Rosacea and Rosacea Treatment

From A Rosacea Sufferer To A Rosacea Sufferer.

Rosacea Tips And Treatment Options

By

Linda Leverston

Table of Contents

Introduction

Growing up, everyone always said that my auburn flame-colored hair and freckles made me look adorable. I always enjoyed these compliments, especially on those days when my mother would dress me up in my Sunday best - a beautiful white frilly dress that complemented my hair and made me look the picture of southern beauty. I felt like a little princess in those days and in many ways I guess I was their little princess.

However, as I entered my teen years, I found myself often teased about my face, which had a blushing tendency. These are some of the most trying times for any young person. You can imagine how embarrassed I would get when the uncontrollable blushing started and I would be around boys. It was mortifying to say the least. Whether this was just hormones playing up or the early stages of rosacea rearing its ugly head, I don't know. All I can tell you is that, thankfully, the following years passed on quietly without much fuss and trouble.

I am married to an amazing and supportive husband who has stood by me through everything and continues to support me in spite of it all. We got married when we were in our mid-20s, the height of life for me at least. We were both fresh out of college, so madly in love and so excited to get started with building a life together and starting a family! We were at that time in life when you are looking your best and the thrill and expectancy of life are just enough to send you over the edge with excitement. That was us.

Fast forward fifteen years, 40 years old and four children later, life has taken a drastic twist. Life is still full of its unexpected joys and little happinesses, but it also can be very ironic, I will tell you that. Sometimes things you never thought would happen will happen and things that you never saw coming will hit you so hard you won't even know what hit you. The truth of the matter is that you just have to get back up when life knocks you down no matter what.

Having gone through the ups and downs of life, my experiences have helped me understand the rollercoaster of emotions people may often face when they go through rosacea. Rosacea can be a very difficult condition to live with, especially when many are not aware of it, and therefore support may not be provided for it. I have read and know of people who have fallen into deep depression because they find it difficult to live with rosacea. They don't have support and because of the lack of awareness, people are not sensitive to their needs. Reading about their experiences makes me sad, but also has pushed me to be proactive. Rosacea does not have to stop you from living a normal life, and this is why I've chosen to write a book about rosacea.

My personal journey with rosacea, as you will discover, is one that has been riddled with moments of pain and triumph as I learned of new tricks to combat the rosacea. It hasn't always been easy, as anyone with rosacea will tell you. But I could not possibly have done it without the amazing support that I found from those around me. So I am going to share a little bit of how I came to find out what was behind the issues with my skin and how I discovered that the frequent bouts of flushing I suffered was actually a lesser-known chronic condition known as rosacea.

My Story

I have always been one of those active moms who attend their children's games. As a family, we are not only social but also very active in our community. My husband played college football and I swam, so getting our children involved in sports was very natural for us. When we got married we never had any intention for our children to be sporty, we just created opportunities for them and encouraged them to follow their hearts.

Those who know me say that I am a very social person and I love being out and about with my friends and family. This is who I am but rosacea changed all that for me…for a season at least… until I got my life back on track.

It all began rather suddenly for me on that fateful morning. It was after my morning run and my face was all sweaty and red. This is typical if you run a lot and I didn't think too much about it. I put it aside and took my shower, but a little gnawing feeling started eating away at me. I almost always know when something is not right. There was a stinging and burning sensation on my forehead, cheeks and face. I increased the water temperature thinking that this would soothe the burning sensation I was feeling, but this only made matters worse.

Stepping out of the shower and looking at my face in the mirror, I was horrified to see that my face was blotched and was swelling up fast. I began to panic and called my husband in. My poor husband must have had a heart attack when he saw my face and I am sure he noted the sense of urgency and panic in my voice. I didn't know what else to do so I got dressed as my husband set up an appointment with my doctor. I am one of those people who believe in catching things as soon as possible before they get out of hand. We don't procrastinate about things; we go to the doctor immediately.

My doctor thought it was nothing major, he said maybe I was just reacting to something I had breathed in on my morning run. I wanted to dispute and say I was sure it was more than that but I didn't know what else to say so I just accepted what the doctor said and agreed to just let it subside with time and take the antihistamine medication for allergies that he recommended. I wasn't aware of any allergies that I could possibly have but I wasn't going to take any chances and took the medicine.

Over the coming days and weeks however, things started to get worse. There were times I couldn't even work on my computer because my eyes began to irritate me. Some of you may have experienced this but it felt like my eyes were dry and itchy or as if I had sand in my eyes. It's the most irritating feeling ever because you obviously can't scratch the inside of your eye!

Additionally, pimples began appearing on my skin. Even as a teenager I had only had the occasional pimple but nothing like what I was now experiencing! My children, who are in their teens, found it a bit hilarious that mom was also getting pimples, at her age! It was *not* funny, I promise you.

Tired of being misdiagnosed I decided to go see another doctor this time. Thankfully, she had an idea what the redness of my face and eye irritation was all about. This doctor had treated another woman who had had a similar condition to mine, so she instantly recognized my symptoms and got me started, fortunately, on some medication that really helped me in those first few weeks. It was through this new doctor that I heard of Rosacea. It was something that I had never heard of before but was so glad to finally have a name after diagnosis so I could do more research in my own time.

For a while the rosacea behaved itself and life continued as normal. The flare-ups only seemed to come and go and sometimes my face would be perfectly normal. At this time I thought rosacea was something that only came temporarily and would disappear with time; I wasn't aware yet that it was something I was going to have to live with and learn to manage for the rest of my life! Such was my oblivion those first few weeks.

After several weeks of carefully managed application of prescribed medicine, I thought the rosacea had stopped, so I also stopped applying the cream I had been recommended by my doctor. That was a bad decision because the rosacea symptoms appeared again and this time with a vengeance! My face was changing. My skin was actually becoming thicker and the pimples that were on my face changed into pustules and began to form on my cheeks, nose and chin! It was horrible and I felt depressed.

I began isolating myself and didn't even want my husband to look at me in my condition. It was too embarrassing and I felt ugly. I have always taken great pride in the way I look and present myself but I couldn't look at my face without cringing, not to mention it really hurt and shattered my self-esteem. Those weeks were extremely challenging for me to come to terms with rosacea. I sympathize with those who are reading this book and have just been diagnosed with rosacea and don't know where to turn to for help or for those who have been living with rosacea for a few years now. I know just how difficult this journey is.

Locked up in my home and too embarrassed to let my friends see me, I turned to the only source of comfort I could think of – online forums. I began looking for answers, anything and everything that was in any way linked to rosacea, I read. I devoured all I could. I bought books and followed homemade recipe options. There was nothing I didn't try. I wanted to find answers and I was impatient!

I even found a dermatologist and went armed with all my information to ask questions and find help. Not satisfied with the answer I got from him, I found another dermatologist and asked the same questions again in case I had missed something. What causes and triggers rosacea? Is it hereditary? Will it end one day? What can I do about it? I think each time they saw my name on the register for appointments they must have rolled their eyes!

They all gave me the same answers, but I wasn't satisfied to just sit back and let rosacea take over my life. I knew there had to be a way to deal with my symptoms effectively. The more I read, the more I discovered that I wasn't the only one out there who was struggling to come to terms with rosacea. It got me thinking. Realizing the amount of knowledge I had accumulated, the time and effort I had spent doing my own research, and visiting countless amounts of doctors and dermatologists, I knew there had to be other people out there who would be happy to have a go-to place to read all about rosacea. This was how this book came about.

This book isn't just about my story but is also about the stories of hundreds of thousands of other people like you and me who have questions that we need answers to. People like you and me who have come to their wits end and don't know how to deal with their rosacea.

In this book, I will share my struggles, my triumphs, my pain and my joy as I continue to live and battle with rosacea. I will share treatments that have helped me and those that have not worked for me but may work for others. I will elaborate on what you can do for yourself to help you live a normal life with rosacea.

Being the social person that I am, rosacea hit me hard and I had to refocus and find a way to continue life, not allowing the condition to stop me or limit me. I had to come to terms with things I could and couldn't do. You will also learn how to support other Rosacea patients and what you can do to get the word out to their loved ones so they know how to treat Rosacea patients.

One of the things that I had to come to terms with was the fact that my family would have to live with me and the way I look. I could have chosen the 'woe is me' path but I chose to live life to the fullest. I didn't want my children growing up seeing their mother suffer and give up. That's not what I want them to take away from this condition. I want my story to inspire them to think, 'after all mom went through she is still as cheerful and as happy as ever, if she can go through that and still manage to enjoy life then there is nothing that can come in our way that we can't face and overcome!' That is the spirit I also hope you take away from this book.

This book is not about feeling sad and depressed about the facts and realities of rosacea. Rather, it is a celebration of what life is about. Let your story inspire someone. I hope that is what you take away from this book.

I want to make special mention of Dr Ruth Randal. She was the star in the midst of it all. She was probably the fifth dermatologist in a long line of depressive gloom and doom doctors. She was like a breath of fresh air because she knew exactly what I was going through. Her own mother had suffered from rosacea and growing up she had seen how it made her mother an anti-social person who retreated from the company of the rest of the world. Her mother's rosacea was so bad that it led her to depression. Dr. Randal's mother's depression was so deep that she never emerged from it and later it sadly cost her her life as she committed suicide. Dr. Randal has given me express permission to include this story because that is one of the reasons she became a doctor, particularly a dermatologist because she understands how illness can affect a person's life and that of their family around them. She hopes that with this book more and more people will be helped and will seek help from the proper channels.

This book is also written to help those who do not suffer from rosacea to understand just what Rosacea patients have to live with. There is a chapter that is solely dedicated to non-rosacea sufferers that will give them advice on how to live with a Rosacea patient.

In the end, I hope this book will be a source of comfort, delivering a message of hope that rosacea doesn't have to mean the end of the world for you or life as you know it. Rosacea is just a stepping stone to everything else life throws at you. Do not let rosacea define how you are going to live out the rest of your days! I have made mention and reference to some of the people that stand out for me who have gone on to do a lot of great things and accomplish big things despite rosacea. I hope that their life stories will also inspire you as much as they did me.

So cheer up and read on to find out the best tips and treatments method around!

Chapter Walk Through

Chapter 1 addresses what Rosacea is. It takes a look at the dynamic aspects of the disease and the common signs and symptoms in adults at different stages of their lives. It also tackles the difficult questions such as, 'is rosacea curable?' and ends with a fun look at some famous faces that live with rosacea. You are going to be surprised by some of them!

Chapter 2 expounds on the common triggers of rosacea as well as trying to explain the cause of the condition. We also tackle the hereditary issue that many people find themselves asking, wondering whether they are like this because of a genetic link and whether or not they are more likely to pass this on to their children.

Chapter 3 takes a look at getting a diagnosis from a physician. There are different doctors who are eligible to treat you. We will take a look at each doctor in turn, from specialists such as dermatologists to those who provide holistic treatment. You may also be wondering how these doctors check to see if you have rosacea or not. This is all explained in this chapter.

Chapter 4 asks the difficult question of misdiagnosis. The statistics of people who have spent thousands of dollars on the wrong medication because of a misdiagnosis is shocking. Before you go ahead and purchase medicine for some other condition, it is good to know what other illnesses are similar to rosacea so that you can be sure before spending any more money on unnecessary medication.

Chapter 5 touches on the challenges that Rosacea sufferers have to live with. It is always good to know that you are not alone in this and that there are solutions to help you live a normal life. You don't need to let rosacea get the better of you. We will talk about treatment options for these challenges in this chapter as well.

Chapter 6 brings you the best treatments on the market. You will learn several new treatments that you potentially did not know of and find comfort in different remedies that are both cost-effective and efficient. The treatments that you will read about in this chapter include treatments that I have tried and some that I haven't tried. The ones I have tried and have been successful with I talk about in more detail and those that I have read about but have never tried are also included. You will also learn the advantages of each treatment and the side effects of each one.

Chapter 7 discusses practical solutions to deal with rosacea as well as tricks and tips on living life as a Rosacea patient. These are the hottest and best tips on rosacea.

Chapter 8 gets into the little details of rosacea. It is common for people who have just learnt about rosacea to be in the dark about some of the not so talked about issues that Rosacea patients face. In this chapter we bring you the good, the bad and the ugly truths about rosacea and how to overcome each one.

Chapter 9 helps you cope with a diagnosis of rosacea. If you have recently found yourself suffering from rosacea and don't know where to go or who to turn to for help, do not be afraid. I know how scary it can be finding out for the first time that rosacea is something you are going to have to deal with for the rest of your life. It's not something you can talk to anyone about. Fortunately, there are places you can go where you will find the help that you need just when you need it. In this chapter we list down all the best places to get this support and help you need.

Chapter 10 addresses the lifestyle issues of rosacea sufferers. Rosacea doesn't have to dictate how you live for the rest of your life. We give you practical guidelines on how to make your life the best one you have ever had despite living with rosacea. This might just be the thing to help you chase your dreams with more passion. I have also included an in-depth look at some of the inspirational people living with rosacea who are doing and have done big things with their lives. If you are anything like me then from time to time you need a little motivation to get out of bed. This is my go to chapter for such mornings!

Chapter 11 is written to help the loved ones of those suffering from rosacea. It is an easy-to-read guide on how to practically help Rosacea patients. It teaches friends and family members how to support their loved ones who are suffering from rosacea and makes them aware of the things that we as Rosacea patients may be too embarrassed or too shy to say in person. It is written in a humorous way that will help others see rosacea as if they were in our shoes.

Chapter 12 "Final Thoughts" just sums up everything that we will have read and learnt about in this book. It brings the books to an end and gives you an overview of the important points that were discussed and mentioned in the book. If you want to skim read the book and get a feel of what the book is about, reading this section of the book will definitely help you to get a comprehensive overview.

Chapter 13 "Frequently asked questions" is a reference section that answers all the common questions about rosacea. It is a useful section that you can always go to, even if you haven't finished reading the book, and you are looking for a quick answer about an issue. It really is a great resource and one that I am sure you will find very useful. I added this part because I understand that sometimes all you are looking for is a bite-sized answer in the moment and don't want to have to read pages upon pages of text to find the answer you are looking for.

The Resource Guide simply outlines useful websites, forums and discussion groups you can join to find help and support. Sometimes if you live alone or don't have anyone close to you, joining an online support group can be a neat way to get in touch with other rosacea patients and find the support you need. What's more, if you find a great community, you will be kept informed about special events and special days where you can meet other people in person and get to know more people in your own area.

CHAPTER 1 - What is Rosacea Syndrome?

Rosacea (which is pronounced roh-ZAY-sha), also known as acne rosacea, is an often misdiagnosed medical condition that typically affects fair men and women of Celtic, Scandinavian and Irish descent as they pass through menopause but can begin earlier in life around the late 20s. Rosacea is characterised and identified by its tell-tale symptoms, which are redness of the chin, forehead, nose and cheeks. It is often referred to as acne rosacea because it can produce minute, red pus-filled pustules on the face that look like those of acne.

Rosacea is chronic, which means that those who suffer from it deal with it for a long time, either continuously or every now and then, when it appears and then disappears for a while, only to reappear again. Rosacea can last for years and is incurable, hence Rosacea patients must learn to live with it and manage the symptoms of the condition.

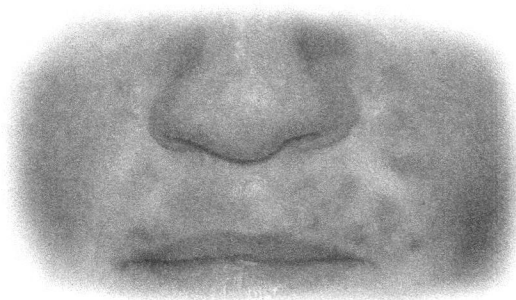

The name Rosacea is Latin and means rose colored or made of roses.

The American National Rosacea Society, which is the largest organization that conducts research and work related to rosacea, states that rosacea can be subcategorized into four main classes:
- Erythematotelangiectatic rosacea
- Papulopustular rosacea
- Phymatous rosacea

- Ocular rosacea

Each of these four classes exhibits common symptoms of rosacea but there are differences between each one, which your dermatologist can identify and prescribe the proper medication that will work for your particular type of rosacea.

We are going to look at the general characteristics that may be used to identify rosacea, and then we will look in more depth at the specific symptoms that affect and distinguish each of the four rosacea subclasses.

Common General Symptoms of Rosacea

Symptoms that are common amongst rosacea sufferers include the following:

Face
- Redness of the cheeks, which resembles flushing of the face
- Redness of the forehead
- Redness of the nose
- Redness in the chin area
- Inflammatory papulopustular rosacea - Pustules filled with pus (sometimes these are simply bumps that have no pus in them)
- Bumps that resemble acne appear on the face
- Small blood vessels that may be visible on the nose. These prominent blood vessels are medically known as telangiectasia and signify the first stage of erythematotelangiectactic rosacea. The area that is normally affected here becomes swollen, warm and has the characteristic redness of rosacea
- As time develops, skin can become thicker as a result. This thickness is usually seen on the forehead, cheeks, chin and other body parts
- Dry and flaky facial skin

Eyes
- Puffy, swollen eyes

- Eye irritation due to dryness
- Eyelids may also become inflamed

Rosacea, like most illnesses, can manifest itself in many forms and carry different symptoms in different people, but the symptoms that are most often recognized as symptoms of rosacea are the ones listed above.

It is not uncommon for rosacea to be misdiagnosed as acne or other similar skin conditions. Other, lesser-known symptoms that often lead to a misdiagnosis of rosacea are:

Face
- Oily skin
- Red rashes
- Red spots that tend to become painful with time
- Itching
- 'Santa' nose – bulbous red nose is commonly seen among male rosacea patients
- A stinging feeling or sensation in the face, which can sometimes lead to swelling of the face

Rosacea needs to be tended to immediately because it can get worse with time if it is not treated.

Your doctor may have correctly identified rosacea using the above common symptoms but in order to find you the right solution he or she needs to now identify which type of rosacea subclass you fall under. These are the characteristics that he or she is going to be looking out for:

Specialized Signs and Symptoms of the Four Subclasses:
(1) Erythematotelangiectactic rosacea
- Flushing occurs centrally on the face and is generally followed by stinging sensations
- The skin is of a finer texture than the other four types

- The face of patients who suffer from this type of rosacea tends to have a rough scale to it
- The triggers that are common for this type of rosacea include hot beverages, hot showers and baths, changes in weather, spicy food, emotional stress, alcohol and exercise
- The rosacea patient complains of severe pain in the event of applying a topical cream

(2) Papulpustular rosacea
- Most people with rosacea fall within this class
- Middle-aged women are the most numerous in this subclass
- There might be a history of flushing by patients in this category
- The redness is generally on the centermost part of the face, with minute papules encompassed by pustules
- Visible blood vessels may exist, but due to the papules they might be difficult to see clearly

(3) Phymatous rosacea
- The skin on the face tends to be thicker on patients suffering from phymatous rosacea
- The face shows surface nodules on the chin, nose, ears, forehead and eyelids

(4) Ocular rosacea
- Inflammation of the eyelids as well as the meibomian glands
- Visible conjuctival telangiectasias
- Blepharitis
- Interpalperbral conjunctival hyperemia
- Conjuctivitis

Once the doctor has specifically identified which type of rosacea you are suffering from, they will be able to then arrange the best treatment plan for you. In general, the doctor will need your medical history to help him or her determine just which type of rosacea you may be suffering from. You may find that it will take a few weeks before you are certain of the rosacea subtype and you may be asked to go home and keep a journal of all the symptoms you feel and experience on a daily basis.

How rosacea affects the eyes

Rosacea typically affects the dermis of the face. It can however have an effect on the eyes, often leading to painful and uncomfortable symptoms. When rosacea affects the eyes, it often leads to eye problems that need to be treated with great care. The eyes tend to change color, with the white part of the eye becoming red and itchy.

It is not uncommon for the eyes to become dry as well and many patients have complained of feeling a burning sensation in their eyes. Other people report that they find it hard to control their tears and find themselves shedding an excess amount of tears. Others complain of itchiness and irritation in their eyes, as if they had sand in their eyes. For me this was how my eyes would feel after I had been out in the wind or the sun.

With rosacea, the eyes are prone to becoming light sensitive and Rosacea patients can commonly experience blurred or distorted vision. When vision problems persist, it is recommended to see a specialist eye doctor.

The common diseases that accompany ocular rosacea include conjunctivitis, keratitis, and episcleritis.

Often rosacea patients have to work with an ophthalmologist to help relieve secondary symptoms brought about by rosacea. Rosacea eye symptoms can all be managed and kept under control.

Which ages are prone to getting rosacea?

Rosacea is a condition that typically affects fair, middle-aged women. Rosacea is rare in children between the ages of 0 and 12. It is also rare in teenagers between the ages of 13 and 18. It becomes very common from the age of 19 and up. Even 60+ year olds are prone to developing rosacea. The age group most affected, however, is the 30 - 59-year-old range of women.

Rosacea tends to be very severe at this age range. I was getting towards 40 when I finally got my rosacea diagnosed, which means that it probably started much earlier but got severe as it went untreated.

Rosacea does affect both men and women alike but tends to be more common in women. More often than not, when rosacea occurs in men, by the time it is diagnosed, rosacea has already done much more damage because men are a bit more reluctant to seek medical attention for it. However, the sooner rosacea is diagnosed in both sexes the better, so that effective treatment options can be arranged.

Who makes the diagnosis?

Rosacea is a dermis problem and can be diagnosed by medical doctors. However, it is not uncommon to get a misdiagnosis from medical doctors, so most people get a second opinion from specialist doctors, such as dermatologists.

Getting a diagnosis for rosacea does not require complex testing or imaging; this will be discussed in more depth in Chapter 3. We will also be looking at potential misdiagnosis cases in Chapter 4.

Is Rosacea curable?

Rosacea is a chronic illness that is sadly not curable. The chronic nature of rosacea means that it is a long-lasting condition that must be managed medically. However, with proper medical treatment rosacea may be controlled and with time your skin can appear much better.

There are many treatment options out there on the market right now to help Rosacea patients live with the condition. In this book we are going to look at several of these treatment options and will discuss their advantages, disadvantages and effectiveness. We discuss both the natural treatment methods for those who would like to take a more pro-natural role in their treatment as well as other, more traditional methods.

Rosacea syndrome statistics

In the United States of America more than 3 million people are diagnosed with rosacea every year. In total, more than 16 million Americans have been diagnosed with rosacea – that's 1 in every 20 people. That is a really high figure! It is thought, however, that there are more people who are misdiagnosed or who don't know they have rosacea, so the numbers could be much higher than officially recorded statistics.

The National Rosacea Society of America, in a survey conducted in the US among those who had recently been diagnosed, showed that more than 95 percent of the rosacea sufferers were not aware of having the condition and had no knowledge of its symptoms. These are the lucky few who actually manage to make it to the doctors and get started on a treatment plan. There are millions out there who are suffering in silence without the prior knowledge of this condition.

In the United Kingdom, 1 in every 10 people suffers from rosacea. That is almost 2, 8 million people out of the entire population.

Celebrities who suffer from rosacea

Many people are going to be surprised to learn who among the famous faces of our time suffer from rosacea. These famous people have managed to keep their rosacea so well managed that when I first read about them, even I was surprised! Hopefully as you read about them you will be inspired to start taking better care of yourself and managing your rosacea better, like I was. So are you ready to find out just who are the most common celebrities that have rosacea? Drum roll please.

On our list we have a onetime president of the United States of America; we also have one of the hottest film stars on the planet and not forgetting a crown prince. Yes, the list is pretty impressive.

The top five run down:

5. Sex in the City actress and American National Rosacea Society celebrity spokesperson: Cynthia Nixon

Cynthia Nixon admits that as the years wore on she suffered more and more, as her complexion was always flushed. She found it highly embarrassing and hated every moment of it. It wasn't until she went to the doctors and she was diagnosed as having a mild form of rosacea that she understood why she was constantly red in the face. Ms. Nixon now keeps her rosacea under control thanks to oral medication she takes regularly. Ms. Nixon has also said that she avoids all harsh facial cleansers and only sticks to gentle cleansers that don't aggravate and irritate her skin. If you look for any press releases from the National Rosacea Society of America, you might be able to hear Ms. Nixon speak about rosacea, seeing as she is their brand ambassador and celebrity spokesperson. Ms. Nixon works in partnership with the society to help raise public awareness of rosacea.

4. Hollywood actress, Renée Zellweger

Ms. Zellweger has been doing well for herself in the Hollywood movie industry and that's not the only thing she has been doing well. The lovely Ms. Zellweger is a poster child for every woman suffering from rosacea; being a Rosacea patient doesn't mean your face is scarred for life. With careful treatments and watchful care over one's skin, rosacea can be kept to a minimum. While I understand that Ms. Zellweger probably has a team of stylists and makeup artists to help cover the rosacea when she walks out on the red carpet, one thing we are definitely sure of is that makeup can only do so much. So if your face isn't looking too good, makeup will not be able to hide it all. In Renée's case, she has always shown us a fresh face and for that we are grateful and we can learn many lessons.

3. Former President of the United States of America, Bill Clinton

While the former President of the United States will probably never outlive the one embarrassing incident that marred his presidential time in office, it turns out that he has yet another condition that he has always been embarrassed about. While you don't typically think of Bill Clinton as the blushing type, rosacea seems to have caught up with him in the later stages of his life if pictures we see of him now are anything to go by. During his tenure as president, Clinton was often seen with the characteristic ruddiness, and this was attributed to the high stress levels that come with being the president of the free world, but now we know that it was indeed rosacea.

2. Mother and son, Princess Diana and Prince William

While Princess Diana is no longer alive, her son Prince William has inherited her characteristic charm and gentleness. He has inherited all the qualities that we would expect from a crown prince, of course, but he has also received a rather unusual characteristic – a ruddy complexion. London Free Press has been quoted saying that one famous face with rosacea is the heir to the British throne Prince William, Duke of Cambridge. Ann Chubb, author of Royal Fashion and Beauty Secret, wrote about Prince William's late mother Princess Diana, stating that the late princess also had rosacea.

1. Hollywood bombshell, Cameron Diaz

Now we all know the stunning Ms. Diaz from her many movies such as My Best Friend's Wedding, Gangs of New York and the Charlie's Angels series. Not once did we ever catch Ms. Diaz looking ruddy or get the impression that her rosacea wasn't under control. She is a model of beauty and has graced the covers of scores of magazines and international publications. During an interview with Parade magazine, Cameron Diaz admitted that her skin suffered constant breakouts, something that is common for many rosacea patients, yet it is so hard to think of Ms. Diaz even having a pimple on her pristine face.

There is no excuse at all for not working on our faces and ensuring that we always show and present our best foot forward when we step out in public.

CHAPTER 2 - The Pathology of Rosacea

As we try to get a better understanding of just what rosacea is, we have to go back to the basics and ask the crucial questions such as what causes rosacea? Or what triggers the flare-ups that are so common to rosacea patients? We have to look at these common triggers and see them for what they are so that we can effectively get over them and manage them.

What causes or triggers rosacea

Doctors, dermatologists and other skin experts are not quite sure what exactly causes the onset of rosacea. The cause is still shrouded in mystery, however this is not to say that scientists don't have assumptions. There are several possible reasons, yet still there remains no concrete or solid evidence for scientists to make a conclusive statement about the exact source of rosacea.

In the category of leading possible causes, we find arguments being put forward for cases related to dysfunction of the immune system, heredity and genetics, and a general propensity towards blushing amid external factors that are associated with being rosacea triggers.

The most common assumption that has strong support is the idea that the characteristic redness associated with rosacea is the result of blood capillaries that are dilated. The dilation of blood vessels is what leads to the red, flushing color and rosiness that is characteristic of the condition. The difference between the blood vessels of rosacea sufferers and other people lies in the fact that the blood vessels of rosacea patients dilate too easily.

Rosacea's pathology explains that rosacea is an inflammatory disease that is chronic.

It is to be noted that the pimples that are seen on the faces of rosacea sufferers are not in any way linked with bacterial infection. Another culprit that has always been believed to be behind rosacea is demodex.

Demodex is a microscopic mite that makes its home on the facial skin of human beings. It was believed that demodex was responsible for rosacea because of the increased numbers of the mites on the facial area of rosacea sufferers. This has now been disproved and demodex, while playing a significant part in the irritation of the face, is not the main cause of rosacea.

Demodex has actually been discovered to be among the useful microbes that live in our bodies. These microscopic organisms help get rid of the excess dead skin cells on our bodies. They're actually really good because dead skin cells are nothing more than waste accumulating on our bodies and hence need to be gotten rid of.

While demodex has not been claimed as the main cause of rosacea, it has been noted that in individuals who are more prone to papulopustular rosacea, the density of demodex mites has been significantly larger than in non-rosacea sufferers – up to 15 – 8 times more. This was observed in the research done in Brussels, Belgium by dermatologist Dr Fabienne Forton et al.

Common triggers

Rosacea has been known to have certain triggers. It is imperative for every rosacea patient to identify their own unique set of triggers that lead to flare-ups, as they can be unique to each individual. Something that may cause one person to react may not affect the next person. Hence, it is imperative to take note and keep a diary to document environmental factors or lifestyle factors that may be behind rosacea flare-ups for individuals.

I like to distinguish the triggers into two main categories:

- Trigger factors that many people have documented about and written about
- Trigger factors that were common in a group of rosacea patients who took a survey carried out by the National Rosacea Society of America

Heat

When it is hot, or when one is in a hot area, the tendency to flush is greater. This also includes when one is in hot baths. Heat has been singled out as one of the key triggers of rosacea. This is because when it is hot, or the body is in a hot environment, internal temperatures increase. In order to make sure that the body's internal temperatures are kept optimum and at their ideal, the body has to find a way to get rid of the excess heat. One way of doing so is to dilate blood vessels so that more blood can flow. Blood vessels that are found closer to the surface of the skin are also dilated. On the face, it is these blood vessels being so close to the skin's surface that brings about the red flushing color that we see.

Heavy exercise

When you exercise heavily there is greater flow of blood around the body and also within the face. The blood capillaries dilate to accommodate the high pressure when you exercise. The faster your heart beat (i.e. increased heart rate), the more your blood vessels must expand to cater to high blood pressure. This can trigger the onset of rosacea.

Sunlight

A survey conducted by the American National Rosacea Society cites exposure to the sun as the leading trigger for rosacea flare-ups.

Staying out in the sun for too long can draw blood towards the face, causing you to flush. The more you are exposed to the sun, especially during the summer months, the more your rosacea is likely to become worse if you do not take good care of yourself. If you have to work or be in the sun a lot, make sure you always walk out with your sunscreen and a hat with a wide brim.

Ensure that you use sunscreen and even incorporate it into your daily moisturizing routine. This is because sunscreen will provide protection against UVB and UVA rays. Never go out in the sun without first having put on a sufficient amount of sunscreen that has a sun protecting factor of at least 15 (SPF15).

Changing seasons

Every season of the year can pose its own set of challenges for rosacea patients. Summer brings its own set of joys, as most people head out to the beach to enjoy the sun and bathe in the cool waters, and winter complete with the cold and wetness can be a somber time. A change in seasons can cause major flare-ups. This is according to a recent survey that was conducted by the American National Rosacea Society. In the survey, 852 rosacea patients were questioned about the change of seasons and the effect it had upon their condition and more than 90 percent of the respondents said that they were affected and suffered with each change in weather. 58 percent of rosacea patients said that their rosacea symptoms were worse in summer.

Wind

Winter and fall can bring about strong winds and a drop in temperature, which can affect rosacea patients considerably because of the sensitive nature of their skin. If you have to go out when it is windy, make sure you are fully wrapped up and your face is protected. Purchasing scarves that you can cover your face with can help lessen the sting of the wind on your face. Don't worry, you don't have to cover your entire face. You can simply cover your nose and cheeks. Wearing a coat with a hood can also be very effective and helpful.

Hot and spicy food and drink

Spicy food should be avoided by rosacea sufferers. Why? Hot and spicy food causes blood to rise up to the face and can cause the blood vessels to become dilated, leading to the characteristic rosacea flushing. This is not to say, however, that you cannot enjoy spicy food. You can always opt for milder flavors, but if you have spicy food cravings, just limit your intake to once in a while instead of all the time.

Drinking alcohol

Alcohol consumption has been known to lead to rosacea flare-ups. Alcohol acts as an irritant when it is circulating in the blood and should be avoided or kept to a minimum. Drinking too much can result in an aggressive rosacea flare-up. Most people suffering from rosacea often find themselves being asked if they have been drinking alcohol when they flare-up. If you are not sure what the exact cause of your rosacea is but you enjoy a glass or two of alcohol every night or every week, why don't you skip the alcohol and see if you still have the flare-ups.

Menopause
The onset of menopause is usually accompanied by the start of rosacea. More and more women suddenly discover that they are suffering from rosacea as they enter menopause. Why rosacea affects women as they enter menopause is largely believed to be because of the change in hormones. This imbalance causes some women to develop the pimples and pustules that are often seen among rosacea patients.

Emotional stress
Stress is often another major trigger for rosacea. In fact, in a survey carried out by the National Rosacea Society of America, stress was the number two most common rosacea trigger. Stressful situations in life such as changes in jobs, children moving in or out of the house, the death of a loved one, or indeed any situation that has the potential to bring about a stressful result should be avoided by rosacea sufferers.

Hereditary
People who are prone to blushing are often more likely to be diagnosed with rosacea in their later years. In terms of rosacea being hereditary, there is no concrete evidence to support the idea that rosacea is genetic. However, if someone in your immediate family has suffered from easily dilated blood vessels, then you might be at a higher risk of also inheriting this tendency. This is seen in our celebrity example of mother and son, Princess Diana Spencer and son Prince William.

There are, of course, many other triggers that have not been highlighted above. The triggers highlighted above are those that occur more often in rosacea patients. People who know of the common triggers usually discover that when they avoid these triggers or cut them out of their lives, their rosacea symptoms do not appear as often. Personally, I have triggers that may not be common to every person, such as when my food has too much salt in it or is too sweet. I am not quite sure why this happens and as such I have not written extensively on these triggers but would like you to know that if you do not find your triggers on this list, it doesn't mean they don't exist. The simplest and easiest test to try to determine if something is a trigger or not is to take some time and avoid that particular thing you think is causing you to flare-up. Observe yourself for a couple of days and then eat or expose yourself to that thing and see if you get a reaction or not. Sometimes it's nothing; sometimes you may discover that it is a trigger.

CHAPTER 3 - Diagnosis of Rosacea

Rosacea, like any other medical condition, is one that most people often seek help with when they notice changes in their skin and bodies that they believe should not be there. This was my experience, as shared earlier in the book. For me it was after one of my morning runs when I suddenly found myself with a flare-up that was getting worse by the minute. I am not one to wait it out and hope for the best, so I got my husband to set a doctor's appointment with our physician immediately. However, I was misdiagnosed and was put on medication for supposed allergies. It wasn't until a few months later that I went to see a different doctor to get a second opinion. It was there that I was referred to a skin specialist, a dermatologist who correctly identified my rosacea.

Whenever there is a problem that needs to be addressed, you should go to see a specialist doctor immediately. The doctor will take you through a series of tests and examinations to determine the nature of the illness at hand. This collection of history and testing is what is known and referred to as making a diagnosis.

The best doctor to visit
Rosacea is a condition that affects the dermis of the face or the skin of the face. Your general GP should be able to diagnose rosacea. However, the best doctor to go to in terms of skin-related issues is a dermatologist.

Dermatologists are specialist doctors whose area of expertise lies in skin, nails and hair. They are the best doctors to go to when you are looking for precise and accurate diagnosis of all your skin-related conditions.

Who else can make the diagnosis?
Sometimes allergy and immunology doctors will be able to make a diagnosis. They are specialist doctors who are concerned with issues pertaining to allergies and diseases of the immune system.

Your primary care providers may also be able to pin point exactly what it is that is ailing you. Your primary care providers are responsible for the prevention, diagnosis and treatment of common diseases.

How is rosacea diagnosed?

The easiest way to diagnose rosacea is for a doctor to make a simple assessment of the state of your face.

He or she will look the common rosacea characteristics, which are:

- Blushing
- Burning in the face area
- Facial flashing
- Small cysts
- Red, pimple-like bumps

The thing with these symptoms, such as flushing, is that many people are not even aware of the fact that their constant flushing might be a medical problem.

There are no specific tests required in order to make a rosacea diagnosis. It is sufficient for a dermatologist to make an observation of your face over a period of time until they are certain of the diagnosis. However, there are cases when a skin biopsy is needed to make a final conclusion on the assumption.

A skin biopsy is a form of testing that doctors use to confirm their suspicions about certain illnesses. A skin biopsy is when a section of skin is removed in order to be examined further under a microscope in a laboratory. Biopsies are not a form of treatment in and of themselves. They are simply a way of further testing and helping give a thorough diagnosis. They are not meant to hurt so don't be afraid of biopsies!

When will the doctor order a skin biopsy?

Your dermatologist or GP might order you to have a biopsy taken when they notice a growth or a pimple changing shape or color. The biopsy is not a standard test for everyone but can be recommended by your dermatologist when they want to further understand the nature of your skin ailment.

How will the biopsy be carried out?

If you are fearful that it might hurt, you shouldn't be. There are several techniques that are used to obtain the skin from your face. The technique used depends on the situation at hand. It shouldn't hurt because you will be given a local anesthetic to apply on the area before the biopsy is taken. The area will become numb so you should not feel anything as the process is happening.

The different types of biopsies that may be carried out by your dermatologist include:

- **Punch biopsies**
  Simple in nature and involve a cylindrical piece of tissue being taken from the area of your face that has the pertinent rash or problem.
- **Shave biopsies**
  Only a sliver of the dermis is shaven off to be studied further in a lab under the microscope. You shouldn't even feel anything with this one.
- **Excisions**
  While these are rare, they are not uncommon. Excisions are deeper and tend to generally cover more area and are intended to remove the unusual parchment of skin completely. These are sometimes not referred to as biopsies because their goal is to remove the problem area entirely. The pain from an excision can be felt days after the procedure, which is why you can request pain relief medication, but it is not usually required.

How is the sample examined further after the biopsy?

The skin sample is kept in a cultured solution and sections of it are removed in order to study them further. Each piece that is cut off is mounted onto a microscopic slide and each slide has a staining solution applied to it to make it easier for the dermatologist to view the skin and any unusual changes. The dermatologist or pathologist (a doctor who has specialized in disease-causing organisms) examines your skin sample and within 48 hours you should have the initial routine biopsy results.

If rosacea is correctly identified at its onset, then a proper and efficient treatment method can be started by the patient. When rosacea is left untreated, it can become worse over time. This is why patients as well as the medical community are pushing for more awareness and public knowledge of rosacea, so that diagnosis can be made more promptly to ensure the health of the patient as well as support for the patient, both medically and socially. Like most medical issues, the right treatment in a timely manner is key.

CHAPTER 4 – Misdiagnosis?

Rosacea and its symptoms can be easily misdiagnosed by a general physician. This is why it is important to seek the services of a dermatologist. This, at least, was my experience. After a few months of taking antihistamines, it didn't take me long to figure out that I wasn't reacting to anything that could potentially be an allergy. I was almost 40 years old and I didn't have any known allergies. I knew I had to get a second opinion so I went to see another doctor who advised me to go see a dermatologist. I followed his advice and went ahead and set an appointment with a dermatologist, who confirmed that indeed I wasn't having an allergic reaction but was rather going through menopause-related rosacea. That was the first time I had ever heard that word, rosacea, the word that would turn my world upside down momentarily.

When a dermatologist does the first standard check-up to try and see what may be causing you to have these flare-ups, he or she will try to eliminate all other causes for your skin issues to ensure a correct diagnosis. As we have seen in the previous chapter, the most common way for dermatologists to give a diagnosis is by simple observation of the skin and when further tests are required they can order you to have a biopsy done.

A case of rosacea or is it just a simple mite infection?

Among the tests that dermatologists perform to eliminate the chances of misdiagnosis is skin scrapping. Skin scrapping is a non-invasive test that is performed right there in the doctor's office that is used to see if the cause for the skin irritation is not a skin mite. These pesky skin mites called demodex are the culprits in a condition that exhibits symptoms similar to those of rosacea. In fact, these mites can trigger the onset of rosacea.

The condition that these mites cause is not rosacea, however. The skin of rosacea sufferers does contain more demodex mites than the skin of other people who don't suffer from rosacea. So being able to distinguish between a case of mites and rosacea is important. A skin scrape will help the dermatologist get to the bottom of it and tell you whether it is rosacea or just a simple mite infection.

Staph infections mistaken for rosacea

Staph infections are caused by the Staphylococcus group of bacteria. When this bacterium congregates, it tends to form little bumps that are filled with pus, similar to those of rosacea sufferers. These bumps are painful and become red and swollen, making it easier for a misdiagnosis to occur. The bumps that occur need to be accurately diagnosed as not being the result of either staph infections or herpes. Sadly, many people have been misdiagnosed because of the similarities that lie in these conditions.

Herpes mistaken for rosacea

Herpes can also cause angry, pus-filled blisters to break out on the face. These too need to be correctly identified in order to be treated properly and not misdiagnosed. Normally herpes will occur around the lips and chin area and will affect mostly these areas. Dermatologists should be able to pick this up easily.

Lupus mistaken for rosacea

Blood tests are not normally required for everyone but there are times when a dermatologist needs to check if you are not in fact the victim of systemic lupus or other autoimmune diseases. Lupus is an autoimmune disease that also causes flare-ups in areas that include the face. One of the major distinguishing features of lupus is that the flaring up is not just in the face but also occurs in other parts of the body tissue, whereas with rosacea the flare-ups generally occur in the face area only. A simple blood test will enable the doctor to be certain about the cause of your flare-ups.

Are there other rosacea look-alike conditions out there?

Frustratingly, yes, there are quite a few rosacea look-alike conditions that really make it harder for dermatologists to accurately make a diagnosis. Rosacea is simple to identify but it might easily be mistaken for another look-alike condition. There are several conditions that may be confused with rosacea, which include:

- Irritant Contact Dermatitis
- Rosacea fulminans
- Perioral dermatitis
- Steroid Rosacea
- Acne Vulgaris
- Seborrhoeic Dermatitis
- Eczema
- Impetigo
- Carcinoid syndrome
- Reactions to medication such as niacin
- Allergies
- Allergies that affect the eyes

Irritant Contact Dermatitis

Irritant contact dermatitis is a condition of the skin that appears as swollen, red, blistering bumps, which may be very itchy. Irritant contact dermatitis is caused by overexposing the skin to irritants such as water, solvents, acid, adhesives, alkalis, detergents and friction to the skin. These irritants then in turn cause the blistering of the skin.

Rosacea Fulminans

Rosacea fulminans is a skin condition that typically affects young women entering adulthood. Young men are not subject to this condition. It is also known as pyoderma faciale. This is a rare condition but when it does occur it produces unsightly and large, red, angry bumps that are quite painful. The area around this tends to be quite red, and the areas affected are the chin, cheeks and the forehead. When comparing typical rosacea with rosacea fulminans, we discover that rosacea fulminans doesn't have flushing as one of its symptoms and neither does it affect the eyes. These two points are what can be used to help distinguish typical rosacea from rosacea fulminans.

Perioral Dermatitis

Perioral dermatitis is more common than rosacea and often presents symptoms in the form of clusters of red, itchy papules around the mouth area. These papules develop towards the cheeks, progressing from the chin area. If a patient is suffering from perioral dermatitis and begins to use topical steroid facial creams, their perioral dermatitis may progress into steroid rosacea. What differentiates perioral dermatitis from rosacea is where the red papules occur. These red papules can go on to occur around the genital skin area and also the anus. With rosacea, however, the symptoms are confined to the area of the face only.

Steroid rosacea

The use of steroid creams on the face can bring about a condition that produces symptoms similar to those of rosacea. The condition that then results is called steroid rosacea because of how strikingly similar the symptoms are to those of rosacea.

The symptoms of steroid rosacea appear on the mid-part of the face, targeting the area around the nose and cheeks. This area will increasingly become red.

With time, acne-like small bumps called papules can be seen and then later on bigger bumps called pustules can start occurring. The ruddy areas often feel like they are on fire and one always feels the need to scratch these reddened areas. These symptoms, as you can see, are so similar to those of rosacea that if not properly diagnosed it is easy to see how one can mistake this condition for rosacea. One way for a dermatologist to rule out steroid rosacea is to check your history and you might find yourself being asked about the topical creams you have been applying on your face.

Acne Vulgaris

It is very easy for rosacea to be at first misdiagnosed as acne. However, further examination of the symptoms can easily help you and the doctor to distinguish between acne and rosacea.

The red spots (pustules and papules) that accompany rosacea are shaped like little domes and not like the pointed spots of acne.

Furthermore, these rosacea spots do not contain blackheads, nodules or whiteheads, as do the spots of acne. These last factors are what can help you to check whether it really is rosacea or just a case of acne.

Serborrhoeic dermatitis

Serborrhoeic dermatitis is a long-term skin condition that is also among the more common rosacea look-alike conditions. It can affect anyone, even infants. This is the very first point that makes serborrhoeic dermatitis different from rosacea because rosacea is rare in children and only appears in men and women entering their late adult life. Serborrhoeic dermatitis is a form of eczema and it affects the face and the scalp areas. Both adults and infants can suffer from this skin condition. It is not uncommon to find, however, that those who suffer from rosacea as their primary skin condition will more often than not also suffer from serborrhoeic dermatitis as a secondary skin condition. The cause of serborrhoeic dermatitis is unknown.

Thanks to the tests that can be performed nowadays and increased knowledge from the research being conducted, there is less chance that rosacea can be misdiagnosed. The sooner you know what you have, the sooner you can start your treatment program.

You as the patient have to work hand-in-hand with your doctor so that you can find out what is behind your symptoms. Don't hide important medical history even if you may be embarrassed to talk about it in front of your doctor, remember that they are only there to help you get better. Some topical creams people use are ones that they often feel embarrassed about or admit to using. Just remember that your doctor is not there to judge you but to offer solutions that will make you better.

CHAPTER 5 - Common Challenges Faced by Rosacea patients

Rosacea patients find that, apart from the flushing they have to live with, there are also facial challenges that accompany rosacea. Two of the greatest challenges are eyesight problems as well as nose related problems. Both issues, if left untreated, can lead to secondary problems, which are harder to deal with. Hence, the sooner these primary problems are dealt with, the sooner a treatment plan can be charted out and planned for the rosacea patient.

Eyesight Problems

Apart from the common areas that it typically affects, such as the forehead, cheeks, chin and nose, rosacea can affect the eyes. When rosacea gets to the eyes, it is known as ocular rosacea. It is important to point out that ocular rosacea does not affect every rosacea sufferer, but it does occur for some and when it does it needs to be identified early on in order for effective treatment to begin.

- **What ocular rosacea does**
  Ocular rosacea is reported in at least one half of all rosacea suffers. So this means one in two people living with rosacea will likely face this problem. Put another way, as many as 8 million Americans suffer from ocular rosacea and up to 1 million people in the UK. The symptoms that accompany ocular rosacea are dry eyes, burning sensations in the eyes, and irritation of the conjunctiva (i.e. tissue that lines the eyes). Some people have reported feeling like they have sand in their eyes. The eyelids can also swell and feel firm to the touch, a condition known as blepharophyma. Others have also had to deal with swollen eyelids, which leads the to eyes becoming sensitive to light.

You should never dismiss signs when you feel your eyes becoming irritable, swollen, itchy or dry because in the event that you leave ocular rosacea untreated for too long, it may bring about harsher consequences such as scarring and damage of the cornea (rosacea keratitis).

All these irritations are part and parcel of some of the challenges faced by people living with rosacea.

- **When is ocular rosacea most common?**
  Ocular rosacea is most commonly experienced when the seasons are changing, whether it is from summer to autumn, or winter to spring. More than 58 percent of rosacea patients find themselves paying the ophthalmologist a visit during this time of the year.

  Ophthalmology chairman at the Northwestern University Dr. Marian Macsai says that 17 percent of all ophthalmic checkups are due to people suffering from dry eyes. This is most common during the winter period because of the dryness that is found in the environment and typically affects rosacea patients.

- **Common treatment options for ocular rosacea**
  When it comes to your health as a person living with rosacea, always be mindful of the smallest irritations, no matter what they are. If you feel any discomfort in your eyes, the sooner you go to see the ophthalmologist the better.
  Many people are quick to dismiss any discomfort they feel and often it is their doctor who picks up on these telltale signs.

  The best way to keep ahead of any potential eye problems is to have regular checkups with your doctor. If anything is amiss, he or she will be quick in referring you to a specialist eye doctor who can perform a thorough routine eye evaluation. If this ophthalmologist discovers anything amiss, they will be able to help you with the best eye care possible.

The most common form of treatment for ocular rosacea is prescription rosacea eye drops.

Nose Challenges

Nasal challenges mostly affect men with rosacea. When rosacea affects the nose, it often causes those who suffer from nasal rosacea to become highly embarrassed and socially shy because of their appearance.

- **What rosacea does when it affects the nose**
  The nose becomes bumpy and red and sometimes dilated blood vessels are noticeable. At times it is the pores of the nose that become prominent; a condition known as sebaceous hyperplasia. If nasal rosacea is not dealt with early on, it may lead to disfiguring of the nose completely, whereby fibrous thickening occurs - a condition known as rhinophyma.

  Rhinophyma is typically referred to as "Rudolph the Reindeer nose" because the patient has a large, red, bulbous nose complete with puffy cheeks. Some people go on to develop bumps on the lower part of the nose and on their cheek areas as well.

- **Common treatment options**
  When rhinophyma is left untreated, one might have to undergo reconstructive surgery of the nose in order to rectify and correct the damaged nose. In general, rhinophyma can be corrected and treated with success by a plastic surgeon or a dermatologist. They will reshape the nose through the surgery. If they don't perform surgery, they will make use of a carbon dioxide laser.

Both of these problems do not need to reach extreme stages. The earlier you visit your doctor with a concern, the sooner you can find a solution and treatment for your problem. Things can quickly get out of hand when you leave them untreated for too long. I have made it a personal priority that whenever I am worried about something, no matter how small, I go see my doctor.

CHAPTER 6 - Common Treatments

We have now established rosacea as an incurable chronic skin condition that will require efficient and effective management in order for it to be kept under control. There are various treatment options on the market; both traditional prescription medicines as well as non-prescription over-the-counter medicine. We are also going to look at natural treatment options for those who are unwilling to become dependent on pills and creams for the rest of their lives. I will present each treatment option as I have researched it and studied it so that you can confer with your doctor and come up with the best plan to manage your rosacea for yourself. I believe it is always good to be knowledgeable about your options and to keep your mind open to other treatments that others are using.

We also know now that simply ignoring the rosacea is not going to make it go away. In fact, ignoring rosacea and choosing to act like it doesn't exist only means that it gets worse over time. As we have seen in Chapter 5, if left untreated rosacea can develop and cause scarring that is both unsightly and painful. The best way to avoid this is to simply work with your physician to develop a long-term rosacea management plan that best suits your lifestyle. Looking after and managing your rosacea doesn't have to be expensive, as you will see below.

Let's take a quick look at the common treatments available before we discuss them in further detail.

Overview of the common treatment options for the face:

- Antibiotics that are topical can be applied to the face. These topical gels will help reduce the swelling of the blood capillaries in your face.
- Some antibiotics come in the form of tablets or pills, which can be taken orally.

- Electro surgery is an option that will set you back a couple of hundred dollars but it is effective when it comes to getting rid of small red lines that can appear on your skin.
- Laser surgery is favored by some rosacea patients because it removes red lines without causing much damage to the skin
- Rosacea sufferers who feel that their nose has become too large may opt to get the extra skin tissue removed in order to reduce the size of the nose.
- Probably the fastest and easiest way to combat and fight the flushing of the skin is to use make up that has a yellow tint to it. It tends to hide the red effectively.

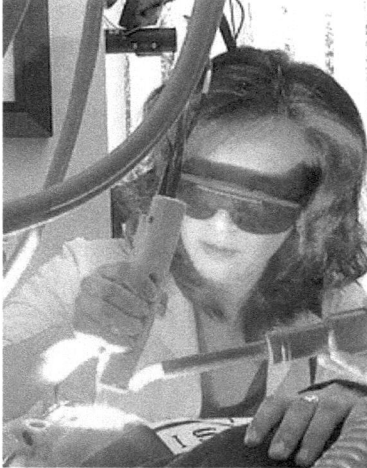

Rosacea Laser treatment. Source: Wikepedia.org

Overview of the common treatment options for the eyes:

- Eye problems in general need the attention of an optician or an ophthalmologist.
- Those who suffer from infected eyelids will have to have their eyelids washed out regularly by their doctor. This is normally done using diluted baby shampoo or a respective eyelid cleaner. After the eyelid scrubbing, a warm compress should be placed over the eyes gently at least three times a day.

- If the eye problems persist or get worse, your doctor may start you on a series of steroid eye medication.

Although we are aware that rosacea has no cure, it still does not stop us from investigating different claims that have been made about treatment methods and options out there. I have scoured the web in an effort to find out all the best kept rosacea treatment secrets people use. Some of these I have tried myself and they have been effective, while some other treatment options did nothing for me. What I hope is that you will be able to discover some new treatments in the following pages, ones you may not have ever considered. Now you can give them a try and see what happens.

On average, when I tried a treatment method, I would stay on that treatment method for at least a month, tracking my progress to know whether or not the treatment was actually working and worthwhile. When a treatment was favorable and appeared to be doing great things for my skin and appearance, I would keep at it until it had become part and parcel of my usual skin care routine. This is one of the key things about living with rosacea and learning to manage it. You have to find something that works for you and stick with it.

The reason why so many people feel frustrated with the treatment options on the market right now is because they cannot stay with one option for long enough to see results. If you are constantly changing medication and lotions, you will not be able to see what is working for you and what is not.

Lastly, you should always follow your doctor's prescriptions and orders. Don't add anymore to the list of medication you have been given by your doctor without consulting with them first. Do not try and self-medicate. I used to be guilty of that. I go online a lot and read scores of articles that have been written by 'rosacea patients' but much of the advice that is given on these forums and pages must be taken with a pinch of salt.

This is why, after much research and editing, I am able to propose and put forward the following treatment options for you.

Oral antibiotics that are commonly prescribed include:

Tetracycline

Tetracycline is an oral antibiotic. What this means is that it is ingested and works against bacteria that causes the acne-like symptoms that we see in rosacea patients.

Tetracycline is great for combating acne flare-ups that are associated with rosacea. This is because rosacea acne and the rash that appears on the face are believed to be caused by bacteria. This antibiotic fights against this acne-causing bacteria. So if you are looking for an antibiotic that will help with the inflammation and the swelling of rosacea, you should have your doctor prescribe you the tetracycline line of antibiotics, which include doxycycline and minocycline.

These types of antibiotics are generally prescribed for 2 to 3 months (6 to 12 weeks) at any given time and the dose will be dependent upon the severity of the rosacea. There will likely be a need to keep getting them prescribed, as these antibiotics do not cure the rosacea but only help to minimize the symptoms of the disease.

The downside of tetracycline is that it does nothing for the ruddiness and flushing of rosacea.

When rosacea symptoms are becoming a little bit difficult to handle, a stronger, more potent dose of oral antibiotic might be recommended in the form of cotrimoxazole or metronidazole.

Sometimes you might wonder why the doctor keeps you on the same antibiotic when you may have read up about stronger antibiotics out there. The truth of the matter is that when your doctor keeps you on the same antibiotic he or she is trying to avoid your body developing a bacterial resistance, which will later hurt you in the event that your body is under attack by a bacteria but none of the medication is working because your body is resisting it. This is why you will be kept on low antibiotic doses of between 40-50 mg doxycycline taken on a daily basis.

Erythromycin
Erythromycin is another great oral antibiotic that can be prescribed by your doctor to fight against acne-causing bacteria. Just like tetracycline, the major downside to erythromycin is its inability to fight off the red color that is so common to rosacea patients.

If you do not particularly like ingesting pills, then there are other ways of taking antibiotics. One alternative way of taking antibiotics is by using topical medicines.

Topical Antibiotic creams that are often prescribed include:
Topical creams that can be applied to the face are popular among both men and women. One such popular topical cream is Metronidazole.

Metronidazole
Metronidazole is an antibiotic cream that can also come in the form of a gel. The advantage that this topical cream has over oral antibiotics and almost all topical creams have over oral antibiotics is the fact that they help more with getting rid of the redness of the face.

There are three other common antibiotic topical creams that are used, which are azelaic acid cream, ivermectin cream and brimonidine gel.

- Azelaic acid lotion or cream – best used to treat mild inflammatory rosacea. It is administered everyday by applying on the areas concerned two times a day.
- Ivermectin cream – a new topical cream that came out in Decemeber 2014. It is used to treat papulopustular rosacea (red bumps that are filled with pus that can be sore). Ivermectin cream is also believed to help with keeping demodex mites under check as well as acting as an anti-inflammatory agent.
- Brimonidine gel – the ruddiness of the face is effectively taken care of by this gel. Brimonidine gel aids greatly with the narrowing of the blood vessels, hence allowing the ruddiness to diminish but when it comes to telangiectasia

(protruding blood vessels), brimonidine gel does nothing for this condition.

Using the two, oral and topical antibiotics, can help to effectively minimize the effects of rosacea greatly.

In the event that you need something else other than antibiotics because your body is not responding well, your doctor might recommend oral isotretinoin.

Isotretinoin
Oral isotretinoin should be taken in minimal doses long-term by rosacea patients. Isotretinoin is a common medicine for those suffering from acne. Like with any medication out there, isotretinoin might not be for everyone, as there are very grave side effects with this drug.

If you are looking for medication to aid with the flushing then you might find yourself prescribed one of the following:

Nutraceuticals
Nutraceuticals are great for reducing the redness that we face and battle on a day to day basis. They are also effective when it comes to reducing the inflammation of the face. I think by now you have picked up on the fact that I suffer from constant flare-ups a lot since my diagnosis and furthermore, being the outdoors kind of person that I am, there is nothing I can do really but continue to look for as many anti-inflammatory and anti-flushing products as I can. Since my first use of nutraceuticals, I have never looked back. They are one of my favorite go-to products when I have a major flare-up.

Within this large family of nutraceuticals you will find a range of medication from clonidine and carvedilol. They both work at reducing the widening of the blood vessels in the face, which leads to the reduction in redness.

The only downside that I have with nutraceuticals that makes me a little reluctant to depend on them whole heartedly is that they cause my blood pressure to drop, which is not good. Sometimes I do experience stomach upsets. Upon conferring with my doctor, I was informed that a common side effect of the nutraceutical drugs is gastrointestinal problems.

Other side effects that accompany nutraceuticals that I have read about but have not specifically experienced myself include the drying out of eyes, a decreased heart rate as well as vision that is blurry.

In my research I came across several other anti-inflammatory agents that other people have used to help treat their rosacea. I will mention these below now, but I wish to let you know that I have not used any of the following medication to deal with my own rosacea and once again, before you decide to start a new course of tablets or creams please check with your doctor to see if they would recommend them to you. Never try to self-medicate but always seek professional guidance when it comes to starting and stopping prescription medicine.

So here are the anti-inflammatory agents that have been used by others to help deal with rosacea.

Oral non-steroids

Oral non-steroids, which include diclofenac, have been known to decrease the ruddiness and general uneasy feeling of the area that is affected by the rosacea.

The side effects of these anti-inflammatory non-steroids include poisoning of the kidneys, hypersensitivity effects and stomach ulceration.

Other anti-inflammatory creams used include calcineurin inhibitors – e.g. the ointment known as tacrolimus and the cream called pimecrolimus.

But that's not all when it comes to treatments. Sometimes, prominent blood vessels can appear on the face and one may feel the need to get these removed. Fortunately, there are two main ways that you can go about this. You can choose to go for either laser therapy or have electro surgery performed on your face. Both are relatively safe.

Vascular Laser treatment

When blood vessels start becoming visible on the surface of the skin it can become quite unsightly. This condition, known as telangiectasia, is the leading cause of vascular laser therapy among rosacea patients. The vascular laser therapy doesn't completely eliminate the visible blood vessels but helps to considerably reduce them.

There are several types of laser available that can help minimize the effects of broken veins and these include alexandrite laser, pulsed dye lasers (PDL), Nd: YAG, Krypton, copper bromide and KTP lasers as well as intense pulsed light treatment.

In general, you should start to see changes and improvement to the skin after two weeks. Regular treatment will help to maintain the results of the laser. When you go in for the treatment you will not be given an anesthetic or sedated because it really isn't required, however you will feel slight discomfort during the treatment.

After the initial treatment you may see a bit of swelling and bruising, but it will disappear and subside within a few days. Should you wish to hide the swelling under make-up, it is perfectly safe to do so. If you can, take a few days off to rest.

When you use the intense pulsed light therapy (IPL) you will find that the therapy itself is very simple. It is neither invasive nor ablative (meaning it does no damage to the top layer of skin). All that is used are high intensity pulses made of visible light that help to make one's skin look better.

Both pulsed light therapy and laser treatments work on the same concepts that make use of light energy. The light energy is absorbed by the target cells containing color found in the skin. After conversion to heat energy, this heat energy destroys the targeted area.

When you schedule your IPL therapy, all you need to remember is to stay out of the sun in the days post-treatment. The treatment session generally takes only 20 minutes and all you need is about 4 to 6 sessions repeated every 3 to 6 weeks in order to get rid of the blood vessels that are causing you discomfort.

It is important to mention that you must always use the services of a registered and qualified IPL therapy agent. During the treatment you should always be wearing eyewear to protect your eyes as well.

The only side effects to these laser treatments include slight pain during the therapy sessions that has been described as feeling like someone is snapping an elastic band on the target area. You might see some swelling and redness straight after the procedure, but this will subside in a couple of hours to days.

In the event that there is neither vascular laser therapy nor intense pulsed light therapy available, you can opt for electro-surgery, cautery and sclerotherapy. Sclerotherapy simply involves receiving injections with strong salt solutions in them.

Electro surgery

Electro surgery is generally used to help get rid of skin growths that are unwanted. The process involves using a high-frequency current that is alternating between voltages of 200 – 10, 000V. This current is then directed into the skin and generates heat that is used to get rid of the unwanted marks or growths.

It is important to remember once again that you should always run everything you wish to do and try past your doctor to make sure that everything is alright. Never undergo a surgery or change your medication without the approval of your primary doctor. Address all your concerns, queries and questions to your doctor instead of looking for answers online. Remember that many people who write online are not medical doctors and have no training and are thus simply writing from a lay persons perspective.

This typically applies to matters when you wish to try out a new drug or a new topical cream. Confer with your doctor to see if the medication you wish to include in your current program will not affect or interfere with the other medication that you are currently taking.

The treatments listed above are some of the more common ones that you will see when you read medical journals and articles. There are other, more natural treatment options that many people have spoken about on the different forums I have been a part of and have followed over the years. I haven't personally tried each and every one of the following treatments but where I have I will tell you how the treatment affected me.

- **Lemon Juice**

A recent letter from a friend informed me about this little tip. Each evening my friend washes her face with warm water and then she applies lemon juice to it. In my research I discovered that whether you use lemon juice straight from the lemon or from a store-bought bottle, you should be able to get the same results.

The lemon is meant to soothe the inflammation and reduce the number of breakouts. It also reduces the amount of time it takes for you to heal when you do experience a breakout. Using this method can significantly help you cut down on the time it takes for the breakout to clear. So next time you wash your face, consider making use of this natural ingredient.

- **Coconut oil**

Coconut oil is used to treat so many ailments and conditions; from reducing stretch marks pre-, during and post-pregnancy, to soothing sunburn. It is also often used as a salve for chapped, cracked heels. It was a small wonder when I read that coconut oil does help with rosacea and relieves the heat-related ruddiness.

- **Green Tea Ice Cubes**

Green tea ice cubes work in pretty much the same manner that a plain ice cube works to reduce the inflammation. However, I have read that chemicals in green tea also have advantageous health benefits for your skin.

This is how you prepare green tea ice cubes:

Make some green tea and let it cool. Once it has cooled down, take an ice cube tray and pour the cool green tea into the ice cube tray. Once you are done put the ice cube tray back into the freezer and leave to solidify completely. The best time to do this is in the morning as you are preparing breakfast so that at any time of the day when you come back home you can always have access to these handy, redness reducing cubes.

Once they are done and you need to bring down your redness a few notches you can easily sit on a sofa and apply the cubes for up to 25 minutes to your face, or until the redness goes down.

- **Tea Tree Oil & Moisturizer**

One of the common skin irritations that often accompany rosacea is itchiness and parched skin. This is a remedy that has been found by several rosacea patients who were tired of their parched skin and needed a solution. What has worked for others is using a few drops of 100% tea tree oil that is mixed with your daily moisturizer and applied to the skin two times a day, preferably in the morning and in the evening. The relief has been described as immediate and many others have also claimed that their skin is repaired from any damage that may have occurred to it from years of being parched and considerable scratching.

- **Dandruff Shampoo**

Dandruff shampoo has been known to work wonders on scaly skin, especially around the nose and the cheeks. All you have to do to see it come into effect is apply a little of the dandruff shampoo on the respective areas and let it sit for a few minutes. After a few moments you will notice that your skin will be more supple and softer and any redness that was there prior to the application of the shampoo is gone.

- **Dead sea salt**

My rosacea doesn't really affect my nose so I don't have a red nose, but I do know several people, men to be precise, who are really affected by rosacea of the nose. For one man it became such a burden and it made his life really difficult. He is married and has two daughters. At school some of the children used to tease his girls about their daddy's Rudolph nose. He told me that it was one of the most painful things to have to endure, thinking how his children had to defend him in front of their friends. Looking for a solution to try and ease the ruddiness of his nose, he read of others who made use of Dead Sea salt.

This man explained to me how he takes the sea salt and dilutes 2 tablespoons of it into one liter of lukewarm water and then proceeds to soak his face in the salty water. The results - this unusual treatment affords him momentary relief but within a few hours the redness reappears.

- **Cut out the excessive exercise and spray mist while you are exercising**

This doesn't sound like medical advice, but it might be one form of treatment you might want to look into, especially if you are one of those people that exercise five times a week. Exercise is good for the body and cutting it out completely would be counterproductive in other areas of your health. So the best way to go around it would be to engage in less frequent bouts of intensive exercise but make sure that the days you exercise you go gently and don't overdo it. Remember that prevention is better than cure.

If on the other hand you simply cannot afford to cut down and you still would like to exercise at your regular pace, then this is what I suggest you do. You need to exercise in a central place where you can plug in a fan that will be blowing air constantly in your direction. You will also need a water spray bottle that you use to spray water on yourself repeatedly during your exercise. This way you avoid getting excessively flared and you also get to avoid developing any facial bumps that tend to accompany flare-ups.

- **Use a block of ice to cool down the face**

When I am having a really bad day and all I want is some instant relief from the redness of my face, one quick and effective trick that I like to use is an ice block. It's really simple. All I do is hold the ice block in my mouth. Using my tongue I alternate the ice block from side to side in my mouth, holding the ice cube between my gums and cheek. It works wonders, even if it is just for momentary relief.

The story behind how I got to find out about this little trick is rather amusing as you will see. I got to know about this little number while I was sitting indoors at the hotel some friends and I were staying at one summer. I was watching my friends hang out by the pool and wished I could join them. I had been out in the sun and had to come back in as I was suffering a really bad flare-up. So seated inside I ordered myself a drink and it came with ice. I just happened to be sitting across a reflective door, and to my surprise within minutes of drinking this cool drink and playing around with the ice at the bottom of the glass, I discovered that my ruddiness was going down. I didn't know what was causing the temporary relief but I figured it was something to do with the ice. So I went outside for a bit and enjoyed the sun a bit more. When I had another flare-up, this time I ordered water with ice in it. I threw the water away and kept the ice. With the ice in my mouth I soon came to the realization that ice was a very efficient and effective way to reduce the effects of a flare-up. That was one holiday I really played out in the sun!

As you can see, there are a lot of treatments out there, both natural and traditional. You and your doctor will work out a long-term treatment plan that will best suit you and your lifestyle needs. If you want to introduce a new treatment into your existing course, on your next visit to your doctor present your findings and ask the doctor if it's possible for you to introduce the new medicine. This is in reference to you making changes to your antibiotics or other prescription medication.

CHAPTER 7 - Living with Rosacea

As we have seen, rosacea can be managed medically for the rest of your life. Learning to live with rosacea means taking into consideration your lifestyle needs and thinking how best to live your life despite the rosacea. Living with rosacea doesn't have to signify the end of life as you knew it. It just means you have to find a way to still do the things you used to do, in moderation.

In this chapter I want to discuss and address lifestyle issues that concern us as rosacea patients. These lifestyle issues also concern those around us who live with us and those who interact with us. Learning how to live with others despite this condition can be a challenge to you as well as it is to those who have to live with you.

Remember that it is probably also difficult for them because they may not know what to say and may inadvertently cause offense when speaking to you about your rosacea. Knowing all of this will help you to not take offense to people's comments, questions or suggestions when they are intended to simply educate. Ignore comments and continue on your path of living with rosacea.

1. Learn to overlook people's words

People can say the most hurtful and thoughtless things. You cannot afford to hold onto these hurtful things that are said. During my first few days, I took offense at the slightest remarks. 'Oh how red you look!' or 'Are you nervous?' or 'What's wrong, are you feeling alright?' People saying these things probably meant well but just didn't know how hurtful their words were.

With time I learned to look past their words and tried to see the concern behind these words. This doesn't mean that it's always easy, especially when it's a stranger asking you such an intrusive question. Just smile and say, 'Everything is alright, thanks for asking' and move on.

2. Be kind to yourself – and your body

At the start of my journey with rosacea I used to be hard on myself. I would get angry when I didn't see results fast enough. I wanted my skin to clear up and stop blushing, so I tried everything in one go, which was a bad idea. I mixed every kind of medication there was that I could get my hands on, and you can imagine how much harm that did me. What I should have done, looking back now with more wisdom and years of practice, was learn to embrace myself and love myself at every stage that I was in. I should have tried one new medicine or topical cream at a time instead of all different bottles together!

3. Getting diagnosed with rosacea doesn't mean it's the end of the world

When I got diagnosed with rosacea, all I wanted to do was dig a hole and bury myself. I didn't want to talk to anyone, not even my supportive and loving husband. No, I shut myself away from the world and cried. There is nothing like sitting across the doctor as he tells you that this is something that you can't cure no matter what you try. To be honest I really felt like it was unfair. All my life I had looked after myself. I was a celebrated athlete in high school and swam during my college days for my scholarship and even after four children I still took great care of my body. I did everything right so why was this happening to me? It wasn't fair I wept to myself.

I didn't realize it then but crying was the best thing I could have done. I needed to cry, it allowed to me to vent my frustration and anger. It was the start of my journey to acceptance and learning to come to terms with rosacea. Now that I have come to terms with it, my attitude is so much better. After crying I did the next best thing, I talked to someone about it.

4. Talk about rosacea with someone

So once I had calmed myself down, I was able to sit down with my husband and we discussed the way forward. We discussed what the doctor had said about my treatment options because to be honest, my mind froze when he said it was chronic and that I would never be able to get rid of it. Having my husband there was not only good for moral support but also because he was actually listening! So when we started talking about it I realized that he knew more about rosacea than me at the start. Gradually he started helping me come to terms with my rosacea and bit by bit I started to regain my life. This isn't to say that it was all a smooth overnight journey. No, as I write now, it's been a few years since I have known I have rosacea officially and still I need someone to talk to occasionally about it.

This is such an important and key part of living with and dealing with rosacea. This is why I have incorporated forums and chat groups into the list of resources you can find online where you can get help and find someone to talk to. I believe in the power of support groups and I know for one that I couldn't have done it without the express support of my husband.

5. Don't feel limited by all the things you need to do in moderation

Sometimes rosacea can feel like it's taking the fun out of your life because of all the things you cannot do, or should do in moderation. You shouldn't drink alcohol, as it can cause flare-ups. You should avoid spicy and rich foods; they too can cause your rosacea to flare-up. And do take it easy with the exercise. It can all seem so much and so frustrating! I know it did for me. I had to learn that how I looked at these warnings either made it more difficult to bear them or made me feel like I wanted to rebel against them. When I realized that these guidelines had been put in place not to limit me but to give me a sense of control over my life, I started reacting to them differently. I still do feel a little frustrated from time-to-time but in general I have come to see that these concerns exist for my benefit and are not there to limit me but to actually let me live the best kind of life possible with rosacea.

Below I am going to discuss some lifestyle tips that will help you on your journey to living with rosacea. These tips have really helped me adjust to and keep my rosacea under check. They are also some of the best tips that I have narrowed down from hundreds that have been suggested by people all over the world.

Useful Tips

The tips that made the list below are the tips that I have found useful. Many others have also found these tips especially helpful.

1. **Cut out wheat**

   Wheat can be a flare-up trigger for some people. Sugar that is readily found in fruits and wines can be a common trigger for some people and so is wheat. What you need to do is keep track of the food you eat and when you experience a flare-up. This will help you gauge and see if you should be cutting out wheat from your diet or not. Other common sources of wheat that we often overlook are biscuits, breads and cookies as well as pastas. So be sure to keep a diary of all your triggers.

2. **When it's time for fun in the sun make sure you are fully covered**

   The sun can exacerbate your rosacea, this can never be overemphasized. When you go out, make sure you use sunscreen as well as take an umbrella or a sunhat. Wear clothing that reflects the sun instead of absorbing heat because heat can also cause flare-ups. Wear loose clothing or free-flowing materials that allow you to breathe comfortably. While it may be hard for those who enjoy the great outdoors, try and minimize the amount of activities that require you to stand in the sun for too long or that require you to be exposed to the sun for long periods of time.

   If your skin is overly sensitive, make sure you make proper use of a pediatric formulation (which is gentle as it is originally for baby skin) and or make use of a moisturizer that is also mixed in with some sunscreen.

   I recommend using Obagi Rosaclear Skin Balancing Sun Protection SPF 30. It might not work for everyone but it has helped me in thousands of cases. It is amazing at significantly reducing the ruddy color I get on my face when I am out in the sun while also giving me that much needed UVA/UVB coverage.

And lastly you can never go wrong with a sun hat with a wide brim!

3. Eliminate everything that stresses you out, your health is worth fighting for!

Often we let the toils of life get to us and we end up losing ourselves to the pressures of daily life. Stress levels take their toll on our health. If you are a Rosacea patient, then you do not need to be subjecting yourself to anymore stress than necessary. You need to sit down and look at your life. Ask yourself what it is that is making you so stressed out and what can you do to change that? Whether it's a job or a relationship that's stressing you out, make sure to talk to someone to see if you can come up with solutions to reduce your stress.

Simple changes such as incorporating exercise and meditation into our daily routine will see our stress levels being cut down and reduced significantly. Try and find out if you can sign up for a fitness class in your area and get a friend to join you. Finding a way to let go of the stress and simply work out will see your stress levels improving considerably.

Meditation is also a great way to relax. Meditation allows you to stay calm, reconnect with yourself and helps you focus on the important things in life. You will find that you will develop a stronger sense of balance after meditation and that you will worry less about the insignificant things happening around you. The initial days of setting up a meditation habit can be a bit daunting and even challenging for some, but you simply need to push through because you have to remember that your health is worth fighting for.

4. Get rid of harsh facial cleansers

We all love brand name products but sometimes these brands sell products that do more harm than good. When you look at the list of ingredients on your facial cleansers and you see many names you can't even pronounce, that is probably the biggest sign that your cleanser is full of harsh chemicals that you probably shouldn't be putting on your face anyway. Remember that these harsh chemicals contained in these so-called cleansers can irritate your skin, causing your face to actually become worse.

In this regard, you will need to develop a regular cleansing ritual. Developing a cleansing ritual is especially important for those of us who use makeup on almost a daily basis. Dermatologist Dr. Debra Jaliman teamed up with celebrity makeup artist Katey Denno to speak about the benefits of ensuring that your face is kept clean before you go to bed each night and the benefits of maintaining and developing a regular facial cleansing ritual that prevents flare-ups from happening frequently.

Before you purchase a facial cleanser, you need to check to see if it has the chemical compound sodium lauryl sulphate. This is because sodium lauryl sulphate has been known to cause irritation of the dermal layer in rosacea patients. When you purchase your cleansers, look for mild cleansers that have ceramides combined with glycerine or mild cleansers that just have glycerine alone. These cleansers will be much better for your skin. This is because both ingredients (ceramides and glycerine) are known to be gentle for those with skin conditions and they help by removing bacteria gently while also attracting moisture to the skin.

To further help you with getting the best skin possible, Dr. Jaliman encourages the use of a humidifier, as it helps keep skin hydrated. As rosacea patients, we all know how sensitive our faces get. When buying a moisturizer also look for one that contains a noncomedogenic. This is because noncomedogenic moisturizers are designed in such a way as to not clog your pores. Noncomedogenic moisturizers are also encouraged because of their efficiency when it comes to sealing moisture in the skin.

If you are like me and would rather put away all the harsh products and opt for more natural facial cleansers and face masks that have natural products in them, then I have good news for you. There are tried and tested natural methods that have been known to work for decades and two of them work extremely well for me. These two key natural ingredients that I use are oats and avocado. Twice a week I prepare face masks with these two ingredients and spoil myself with a facial, and the result is skin that looks refreshingly healthy and beautiful!

5. Learn these 4 make-up basics

I love the convenience that make-up, especially the tinted kind, affords me when it comes to hiding my rosacea. However, after much trial and error with different products I finally learned which products work for me and which ones I have to avoid like the plague. There are four main make-up tips I can give you here from not only my own experience, but the experiences of thousands all over the world over. Here they are:

- Read make-up labels carefully
  When buying make-up as a rosacea patient, it isn't good enough to simply purchase any old product as long as it's a brand name. As a rosacea patient you have to put in the extra effort to read the fine print (literally!) and make sure that it won't do more harm than good to your skin.

  You should stay clear of make-up that is not noncomedogenic and has oils in it. A second thing to remember is that just because a product happens to be fragrance free does not guarantee that it will be a great product for the skin. It potentially could be, but you have to make sure that it doesn't contain any of the following products:

- o Alcohol
- o Menthol
- o Peppermint
- o Clove oil
- o Glycol acid
- o Eucalyptus oil
- o Witch hazel
- o Salicylic acid

It is quite a commitment to remember all of these when going out to purchase make-up but your skin will thank you when you use the right products.

- It's all about the base
I have read about people applying green base to counter their redness before putting on foundation. The only problem that comes with using this green base is that while you have solved the little red problem, you now have a new color to deal with! You now look slightly green or gray! In order to counter this problem effectively, celebrity makeup artist Katey Denno advises that the best base to use is not in fact a green base, but actually a yellow tinted product, which will cancel out and neutralize the red without giving you any more problems!

- **Swap your powder make-up for <u>mineral</u> make-up**

Mineral make-up is so much better than powder make-up because it helps avoid that powdered look that often accompanies using powder make-up. If you are hoping to look flawless, then powdered make-up is not what you are after. Your best choice when it comes to make-up is mineral based make-up.

I am going to recommend a few products that I use here and I will tell you why I prefer them.

Jade Iredale – when I am looking for the perfect cover for work or social events, this is my go to product. In fact, I always have some in my car for those unforeseen times you have to suddenly go and meet someone.

Vapour Organic Beauty – great texture, absolutely amazing products that help treat as well as conceal problematic skin. How awesome is that?

Alima Pure – when I went to purchase my first make-up kit after being diagnosed with rosacea, Alima Pure was recommended to me by dermatologist. She vowed it would be a good place to start as free samples and tester kits are available for you to try out before you make your purchase. I liked this offer so I took it up and went ahead and tried some samples. This was great because I could find the right shade for me before I bought any of the make-up. I ended up buying quite a lot of Alima Pure make-up kits. I have never looked back. I love this brand.

- Keep the make-up light and uniform
When it comes to the application of your make-up, use a light touch. Avoid a heavy hand that will make the make-up look anything but attractive. Make-up should be light enough to look natural during the day. People shouldn't even have to know that you are wearing make-up. While it's true that many people end up going overboard on the worst affected areas, the truth is you just need a light amount of make-up to do the trick. Too much won't make a difference except making your face look all caked out.

  Apply your yellow base cover and then after it place a modest amount of foundation, making use of a foundation brush. Take a sponge and use it to set the make-up in place to create that flawless look that you are after. (Always clean your brushes thoroughly and keep them clean, otherwise they will breed bacteria!).

If you want to know more about how to apply your make-up properly and which other brands are good for rosacea patients, I have included useful links to recognized websites that have been a great source of help to me in my many years of being a patient.

All the tips you have learned in this chapter should come in handy if you use them. If you use these tips correctly, you are well on your way to overcoming one of the more common problems that we face as rosacea patients, the redness that affects us all. These tips are guaranteed to help you live as normal a life as possible without having to worry that people are talking about your uncharacteristic redness behind your back.

Using the tips found in this chapter, now you know what to buy and what to avoid when you go out to buy your make-up as well. You know which ingredients to look out for, which are good for your skin and which ones are not ideal for your skin. Happy shopping!

CHAPTER 8 – Entering the Rosacea World

I gave this chapter the title of 'Entering the Rosacea World' because that is exactly how I felt when I first got diagnosed with rosacea. I literally felt like I was entering a world that was different from the world that I had been living in all of this time. Everything that I knew suddenly changed and my whole life was turned upside down. When people are first diagnosed with rosacea, it really is like their life has been turned inside out and they have to learn to start living life with a new perspective.

Things that you used to do without thinking about twice you now have to stop and think about. You have to ask yourself questions like, is this good for me? Or will this cause a flare-up? You will need to think of ways to combat rosacea flare-ups or to change your lifestyle.

I don't want anyone else to go through the difficult transition that I went through. This is why I have included this chapter in here for you.

- Get a few opinions first – differentiate between acne and rosacea

My rosacea didn't start with pustules and papules, but rather with the uncontrollable blushing, which seemed to increase based on different things I have now learned to identify as triggers.

Fortunately, my doctor seemed to pick it up instantaneously that it wasn't a case of acne, but sadly I didn't get the correct diagnosis. He thought that I was just having an allergic reaction to something. It wasn't until months later that I went to get a second opinion to confirm and try calm the thoughts I was having that kept telling me that what I was going through was not an allergic reaction.

This second doctor, after listening to my medical history, said almost immediately without hesitating, 'It's rosacea.' I guess I was not the first in his office to get treated for rosacea and hence he was very familiar with it. Of course you all know how I sat in that office stunned and unable to process what he was saying. I denied his words for a very long time. It was also at that time that small bumps started appearing on my skin. Because I had already been told that I had rosacea when I read about the pustules and papules starting, I wasn't surprised. Though I will admit that I had last had a pimple in my early twenties!

If I hadn't known about the rosacea, I would have sworn the pimples had been caused by acne. Sadly for many people, they get misdiagnosed and for several months or even years they could be on the wrong treatment, trying to cure something that is not there. Many people use acne creams, which almost have no effect on papules and pustules.

My suggestion is to get the opinion of three independent doctors before you move ahead. Consult with two dermatologists and one physician and compare what they have said and the different treatment options they wish to put you on.

- Read a lot more

I am pro reading and getting people to be aware of their own condition. I admire the effort that American National Rosacea Society ambassador Cynthia Nixon is putting in to get the public more aware of rosacea through her talks about her own journey living and working in Hollywood as a rosacea patient.

When you read, however, avoid the folly of trying to self-medicate through prescription medicines. If you have been put on a certain course of treatment by your doctor, then don't alter or change your medication based on things you have read online. You need to remember that your doctor is in a better position to advise you on what to do than most online articles, which you should know are written by lay people most of the time, people who are not qualified health experts.

Read so that when you go for your routine checkup, you can propose a new treatment to your doctor and can talk about it intelligently enough. Your doctor should then be able to give you advice on what to do if you are thinking of adding a natural treatment option to your current treatment program.

- Keep a journal of your flare-ups

One of the first few things you need to understand about your own type of rosacea is to realize what triggers it and what causes it. The best way to identify these triggers it to keep a journal where you document all your flare-ups and the state you are in when you had your flare-up i.e. had you just finished a round of exercise, or perhaps had a little alcohol, or just plain old walked in the sun without sunscreen? Whatever it is that is causing you to flare-up, you need to document it so that it becomes easy for you to identify your own personal do's and don'ts pertaining to your rosacea.

Get to know the common triggers such as heat, wind, spicy food, hot baths, and exposure to the sun and so forth. Knowing all of these things will help you get started on your journey to living with rosacea and making the most out of life.

When I got diagnosed, the one thing I wish I could have found was a manual like this very one you are reading that gives you information on rosacea and everything you need to get started on your journey to healing in one central place. The tips you are reading here in this condensed format have come from years of reading and a lot of research online, conferring with doctors and other sources to get what you finally see now. If you follow everything you are reading in this book, you will be able to live life with rosacea victoriously!

This is my hope, if you have just been diagnosed with rosacea and don't know where to start, that this chapter really helps you know what to do when getting started on living your life as best as you can. I also hope that if you are a rosacea patient who has been living with rosacea for a long time, now you have also benefited and learnt something new in this chapter. When it comes to the world of rosacea we are constantly learning, there is no end to how much you can know about rosacea.

CHAPTER 9 – Who to turn to for help

When you first get diagnosed with rosacea, you may go through something that I went through. I am not quite sure how to explain it to people, but let's just say it was a bit of depression. Yes, looking at me on the outside, no one would have known the anguish and the battle that raged deep inside me and the things that I was struggling with. My loving husband had always been there; in fact he has really been my anchor because I don't know what I would have done without him.

When we went to the second doctor's office and the doctor said I had rosacea, my mind froze. Everything within me came to a halt. There is nothing worse than being told that the ailment, the illness that is making you this worried has no cure. I felt devastated. How could you tell me there was no cure?

My mind switched off, but my husband continued to listen and he was the one asking all the questions. I don't remember the journey back home, but what I do remember is that I got home and I locked myself in the bathroom and I cried myself to sleep in the bathtub. I remember it so vividly and I share it so candidly because I want to tell you that there is such a thing as post-rosacea diagnosis depression.

At that time I wasn't even aware of the fact that there was such a thing as post-rosacea diagnosis depression and that I was experiencing it. I only got to learn more about it the more I read and researched. In fact, more than 42 percent of rosacea patients surveyed by the American National Rosacea Society admitted to falling into depression at some stage in their journey with rosacea.

Admitting that you may be suffering from depression is hard for one to do and it is even harder to get yourself to the right doctor to get help but it is a step that should be commended – admitting that you have a problem and that you need help.

I have included this chapter in this book because I realize just how important it is for someone to get help at the right moment if they are to get past their rosacea in order to lead and live a normal life.

I have read threads where people threatened to commit suicide because of the complications they found rosacea brought about in their lives. There are people out there who can be very ruthless and unkind to rosacea sufferers. I know. I write from a place of compassion and wish others to know that they are not alone in their sufferings.

Professor Bill Cunliffe, a leading British specialist doctor in the world of skin problems and co-author of several reports published in the British Journal of Dermatology shares that many people don't understand the full extent to which skin problems, particularly facial skin problems, can result in deep depression setting in for the person concerned.

Dr. Cunliffe spoke about the deep psychological and social effects that many people do not stop to consider about people suffering from skin problems. He said the most common problems he found among those he treated with skin disorders included low self-esteem, employment problems as well as job discrimination. All these challenges Dr. Cunliffe said could lead someone to take their own life - something that appears to be happening at a greater and alarmingly increasing rate among adults diagnosed in their later 20s.

The UK especially has been plagued by numerous accounts of college school students who have taken their own lives on account of problems faced from different skin conditions, which include rosacea. The statistics of the UK alone were enough to convince me to include this chapter because I am sure that someone reading this book will be helped or will be able to help someone else going through a similar battle.

I am going to tackle this depression issue from two angles: firstly from the angle of you as the rosacea patient being depressed and getting the courage to call out depression for what it is. Secondly, I am going to address the non-rosacea sufferers on how they can help a loved one or someone they know who has rosacea and who they suspect might be suffering from depression.

Do you have rosacea-related depression?

As rosacea patients, we all find ourselves disliking how we look more often that we should. Our thoughts, however, can at times turn dark, and cause us to fall into depression. Depression is a serious condition and can lead to a greater threat, so if you are going through a tough time, it is important to get the help you need. Sometimes, all it takes is a conversation with a loved one or doctor to help you pull yourself out of a negative spell. Remember, you can control rosacea. Don't let it control you.

Admittedly, although we can be fully in control of our condition, we all have days where we absolutely dislike the way we look and that is normal for a rosacea sufferer, heck it's normal for any human being to have one of these days. The problem occurs when these kinds of days occur consecutively and frequently without respite. When all you think about is how much you hate yourself and loathe yourself, then we might be facing an issue that needs to be addressed immediately. When these become your only thoughts, then there might be a big underlying problem that needs to be seriously looked into before it gets out of hand.

If you identify with any of these symptoms that I have discussed, then you may need to consult a therapist. You need to know that you are not alone and it's okay to ask someone for help. One thing you should know about depression is that it can be treated.

- Go see a therapist

A qualified professional will be able to guide you on how to deal with the negative thoughts you have and might even help you find a support group so you don't have to feel alone in your suffering. There are many groups that meet in person and not just online where people get together to help each other, share tips and tricks on how to live with rosacea, and basically just be there for one another without judgment. Perhaps this is all you need. So don't cancel going to see someone because you think that going to seek help is a sign of weakness.

- Develop good sleeping habits

Other useful things to do that are likely to help include getting enough sleep. Many depressed people may find themselves unable to sleep and facing sleep problems such as insomnia. You need to aim for at least eight hours of uninterrupted sleep when you are going through this depression phase. Sleep will help your body function properly and you will feel your best each morning when you sleep well. When you are depressed, you may also notice a change in your sleeping patterns. You may find that you tend to sleep during the day and are up during the night. Training yourself to sleep regular hours can help you combat and counter the depression.

- Look into relaxation techniques and engage in them

Put on some positive music and listen to it, or listen to something motivational that gets you happy and in a good mood. You have to force yourself to do this even if you are not entirely feeling up to it. This is why having the help and support of others around you can be a really great thing. Relaxation techniques don't have to be complex, overtly spiritual methods, something as simple as stopping periodically during the day and taking a couple of deep breaths can help you refocus and clear your mind.

- Eat smart, eat healthier

Not only is eating healthier great for rosacea but it's just great for overall health and wellbeing. When your body is receiving the necessary nutrients that it needs, you will find yourself feeling much better about yourself and the negative thoughts will start to disappear slowly but surely. The obvious food choices to make are fruits and vegetables. However, everything should be eaten in sufficient proportions i.e. carbohydrates, fats, fruits, vegetables, drink lots of water and also have enough protein. All of these will work wonders for your skin and you will be in a better place all round.

- Do things you love doing

Combining all of these factors with doing something that you enjoy doing every day is also a great way to getting out of depression very fast. Make a list of your favorite things to do and put it somewhere you can see it easily. Your list may contain anything from reading a thrilling book to watching a comedy show on the TV or maybe just listening to some music. Whatever it is that makes you happy, do that. Schedule time in your day where you just get to do something that you like. Even if this means just setting aside 30 minutes every day, you will be surprised by how much that time can make a marked difference in your mood and in your life.

- Resist negative thinking

This one will require a lot of energy and concentration because thoughts come into our mind sometimes when we are not even thinking about anything in particular. When you are facing depression, you will have to monitor all your thoughts to make sure that you are helping yourself by breaking the negative cycle that keeps repeating itself in your life. A simple trick I was taught by my therapist was to keep an elastic band around my wrist. Each time I found myself thinking a depressive thought, I had to snap the rubber band and that almost always distracted my mind from the thought I was having and makes my mind focus on the rubber band! It was a nifty little trick that always did the job.

The second part of dealing with depression is for people who know someone that is a rosacea sufferer and who is also going through depression. This part discusses how you can help the rosacea sufferer overcome their depression. A supportive friend, a shoulder to cry on, you can help rosacea sufferers beat depression. Being there for the person will mean a lot, take it from me. Your participation in the healing of a rosacea patient is an invaluable role that cannot be overemphasized. I don't know what I would have done without the express love and support of my husband, who stood by me throughout the depression and was always there.

I write it for people who are willing to stand in the gap and be there for the depressed person when they need support the most.

Helping a rosacea patient going through depression

It is not easy to be the one having to watch a loved one with rosacea battle depression. My husband had to live with me while I was in denial about my depression for almost a year, until he finally confronted me about it seriously.

I had never thought of myself or seen myself as the kind of person who could get depressed and yet there I was on our bathroom floor almost every evening crying. The crying didn't make matters any better of course because every night before I went to bed my face would be all blotchy and super red.

What I didn't know was that my husband was talking to several medical specialists and describing my symptoms to each of them. They all came to the conclusion that I was in denial and going through depression. My husband didn't know what to do, so he started reading on how to support a person going through depression and these are the things that worked at least for me and other people that I have conferred with as I did my research for this book.

Those around you need to:

- Speak words of affirmation

I found that when people spoke kind words to me and said nice things about things I may have done during the day, it made me feel much better about myself. I didn't have time to think about all the negative things about myself that I used to waste all my energy on. Speaking words of affirmation really has the power to change and uplift a person in such a powerful way because depressed people are usually also suffering from low self-esteem in that moment of their lives.

- Compliment you when you are looking good

My family had seen me purchase tubes upon tubes of make-up in an attempt to hide my ruddiness. My husband started with the habit of complimenting me when I looked good with makeup and when I looked good without my makeup. He wanted me to feel beautiful with or without the makeup. I found that because someone else was invested in me and saw my own worth and my own beauty even when I couldn't see it, it made me realize something about myself – that I was valued and that if I hurt myself I would bring so much hurt to those who loved me the most, my family. So the take away point here is to affirm the person that is going through depression. Tell them their beautiful; affirm their value and their worth.

- Encourage the depressed person to learn a new hobby

It might seem a bit over the top but getting out there and meeting new people might be one way of helping get a depressed rosacea patient's mind off their own thoughts. Enrolling in a calm hobby such as taking an art class or flower arranging class can help your mind engage and focus on other things. I for one took up art classes and found that when I got there, the mood was very relaxed. Everyone would arrive at the class and after a few pleasantries class would begin and for up to two hours my mind was consumed by the work before. I learned a great skill that I still regularly engage in when I want to unwind. Of course these are not the only courses you can engage in, there are hundreds of classes you can look up for the person along their line of interest and help them make up their mind about a class to take.

- Encourage them to go for a walk

I find that going for a walk really does calm my mind. I used to run a lot in the past but now I tend to reserve the running for my exercise days. When I don't run, I walk. It gives me time to just clear my mind and even if my face flares, I take my walks early morning or towards evening when it is too late for people to stare at me, so I feel safe. I enjoy the walks and find them really refreshing. Obviously when it is cold or too hot I prefer to stay indoors. Encourage people going through depression to go for a walk, better yet go with them! Or take a couple of bikes out and go for a ride together.

- Accompany them to talk to a therapist

This may be the hardest thing that you will need to do; encouraging the person you know suffering from rosacea to go talk to a therapist. Often if you approach and suggest this offhand it can be met with resistance and event resentment. You need to introduce the topic subtly. They might feel uncomfortable talking with you about how they truly feel, but they may open up when talking to a stranger. Help them schedule their appointments. This might require you to have to go out of your way to drive them to and from the venue lest they chicken out and cancel their appointments.

Often they will need support but might not want you in the office as they speak to the therapist. They might just want to know that you are there for them waiting, even if it is just outside the office. Be there, it means a lot to them.

Getting help isn't a sign of weakness but is actually a sign of strength, a sign of maturity that you realize when you need someone else to help you up. Reaching out and getting help can be one of the hardest things for people to do as well. One thing to keep in mind about depression is that depression can be overcome. It is worth fighting to get your life back on track because you are worth it.

For those who know someone suffering from depression, being there is one of the best things you can possibly do for that person. It means a lot to them and you may be the strength they need to go out and get help. Sometimes they might not be able to talk to you directly but knowing that you are there and able to offer comfort is sometimes all that they need.

CHAPTER 10 – A Word of Advice for Non-Rosacea Sufferers

If I could rip out this chapter and place it in the hands of every non-rosacea sufferer, I would. These are the top things that I wish every non-rosacea sufferer knew! This list has been made using some of my own life lessons and things I have read from others. I have received thousands of letters from people complaining to me about the insensitiveness they meet and generally just how difficult life can be when people are not aware of their condition. It is hard enough to have to live with rosacea, but having to explain time and time again to those we live with or work with to not do certain things in our presence can be very frustrating.

So if you know someone suffering from rosacea and have ever wondered what they are thinking, here are a few thoughts for you:

'No I don't have a blushing problem so stop asking me about it!'

Fair and fine my rosacea only developed in my mid-thirties, but that didn't stop some people from jesting and making fun of it when I was around. Sometimes at the office, it was one of those awkward questions that I would get asked and I never quite knew how to respond. This fear of ridicule made me hide in my house the first few months after getting diagnosed. I am a very sociable person and so having to hide in my house was very difficult for me. Then again I didn't see it as hiding, but that's what it was pure and simple.

I didn't have the guts to face people out of embarrassment because I was scared that they would ask me questions. It often became highly uncomfortable if I was in the presence of men and someone would bring up the issue. Moments like that I wished the ground would just open up and swallow me. That was when I learned about yellow tinted make-up. Nowadays, the ruddiness has been toned down thanks to this make-up. So, what I want to tell non-rosacea suffers is, don't ask why someone is so red in the face, it really is none of your business.

Don't stare

Staring has got to be the number one thing I still find very rude and disconcerting. I have personally had lots of children point and stare at me, and while they are children I have learned to look past it. When it is an adult, on the other hand, it does become very rude. More than once I have seen people stare at me and it was like I could read and hear their thoughts. Please don't stare, it makes us doubly uncomfortable.

It really is painful

When people ask me, 'So does it hurt?' and I tell them, 'More than you could ever imagine.' I think that people still find it hard to believe or process that. Yes, acne might not be painful all the time, but that's precisely it. Acne and rosacea are not the same thing. You might think they are but I assure you they aren't. Rosacea, especially when the pustules start developing as well as the papules, can get quite sore. I haven't even gotten around to speaking about the burning sensation that you often feel in your face. It's not a pain that can be fully described, but how about, 'It feels like my face is on fire?'

Our self-esteem sometimes hits rock bottom, don't make it worse

While it is true that no one can make you feel worthless about yourself unless you let them, it still doesn't mean the words don't hurt when they are spoken. Sometimes words are said in passing in the form of a question that we might brush aside as we change the topic quickly but that doesn't mean we didn't hear the hurtful words. 'You should try concealer.' Or 'Your skin reminds me of my teen years – the worst years of my life!' or how about 'Your face sure looks like a beetroot!' Yes, I have heard much, much worse if that is even possible.

My little piece of advice – if you don't have anything nice to say, then don't say anything at all. It's better to leave the words unsaid or question unasked rather than to risk hurting someone with your thoughtless comments.

'Can you not smoke in the car?'

I don't know how many times I have had to travel with people and kindly ask them not smoke in the car or not spray their colognes and perfumes while I was sitting in the car. It is so burdensome for us as rosacea patients because we feel like we are being a bother to everyone around us but at the same time if we do not put our foot down, by the time we leave that car we will be in a rather uncomfortable state. So please, be a little considerate.

The same applies to those who like spraying air fresheners and opening office windows in the middle of winter. Small things like that can appear like nothing to you but to us they are big things that can trigger a flare-up that we would rather not have to deal with.

Selfies, family portraits, group photos, sure we'd love to feature in them, just give us a sec….

I love the modern technology that we have. I love the convenience of going out with friends and family and just enjoying each other's company. It is always lovely until it comes time to take a few pictures – then it gets awkward. Because as rosacea patients we tend to be very self-conscious about the way we look, so please be patient with us if we ask you how we look, or if we excuse ourselves to take a quick look in the mirror. You don't want to be the odd one out in the picture who looks like they had just completed a marathon when someone decided to take the snapshot! It is not vanity when we check in the mirror; it is just to make sure that we are happy with how we look before our faces are immortalized for life!

Rosacea comes and goes

People sometimes bump into me and my rosacea has been clear for a few days and they remark, 'Wow! Your face has cleared up; maybe it's gone for good this time.' You have no idea how much I wished my rosacea would go away for good. Sadly it's something I have to live with for the rest of my life. While it is nice to receive pleasant, positive comments about the rosacea clearing up on certain days, we just wished you didn't have to bring the topic up again when you next meet us and our faces aren't looking as good as they did on that other day!

If you are a close friend and we hang out, don't force us to drink alcohol!

Going out to hang out with the girls or with friends and family can be a struggle when everyone else is enjoying their wine and alcohol. The temptation to drink is already there, especially for those who used to drink but can no longer drink now because of their flare-ups. I know a friend suffering from rosacea who hangs out with friends who all drink. So when they go out for some fun, it's a bit difficult for him to say no. He has relapsed into his old drinking habits and the effects are showing on his skin. He had stopped drinking for close to two years when he relapsed and went back into drinking. In his case, what makes it doubly hard is the fact that he doesn't just drink beer, but also likes strong spirits. When I saw him recently my heart went out to him because his face has suffered, which has in turn affected his self-esteem. My advice is this - if you enjoy drinking and you have one mate with rosacea, try and tone down on coercing them into drinking. They are already having a hard time without you making it harder for them.

Don't stress us out please!

Life gives us enough to stress about as it is so please don't add to all our problems. For women, emotional triggers are often common and so are changes in hormonal imbalance. Emotions and hormonal imbalance are two triggers that can cause flare-ups in women. Many women attest to the fact that as soon as they feel like they are about to cry or to have a stressful day, they feel the flare-up starting and no, it's not pleasant, it is downright painful!

It's hard having people question your personal hygiene when they see pustules on your face

Some people have made themselves know-it-alls and conclude that our pustules and papules are the result of a lack of personal hygiene on our part, that we somehow don't know how to wash our faces properly and take proper care of our skin. I haven't had this personally happen to me but I did speak to a young girl in her late 20s who said all through high school she was teased and bullied because of this very same issue. It didn't make matters any better that she wore braces and spectacles. However, if you see her today, she is the perfect picture of health and indeed should be a rosacea ambassador. Her skin has cleared and looks remarkable, even for a rosacea patient. I asked her what her secret was and she said moderate exercise balanced with a good diet combined with a strict no-alcohol regime. We could learn a lot from this young lady and I really do admire all her efforts to fight and change the stereotype about rosacea and personal hygiene.

No I am NOT drunk and neither am I feeling shy or embarrassed.

I find this kind of insensitive comment very rude and upsetting for several reasons. Personally, I do not drink, so when people see me getting flushed it is always disconcerting to have people assume it is because I have had one too many to drink!

Even for those who do drink, they find it very rude when people ask them if they have been drinking simply because they appear a bit flushed.

The second kind of comment that really annoys and ticks a lot of rosacea patients off is when people ask them if they are embarrassed or feeling shy about a particular matter. What people need to understand is to simply mind their own business when it doesn't concern them instead of making ignorant and hurtful remarks.

You haven't seen me out and about because perhaps I have been trying to avoid these kinds of questions.

Sometimes people approach me and ask me why they haven't seen me out and about at social events or at gatherings. One thing about rosacea is that it can get quite debilitating when it decides to be troublesome. Sometimes I find that the effort I would need to put in covering up the redness with layers of make-up is simply far too much and I would rather just kick off my shoes and stay indoors.

Some of my closest friends are those who now understand that when they don't see me at social events, it's not that I don't want to go but it's probably because that day I am having a really bad case of flare-up.

This isn't to say that as rosacea patients we should keep ourselves hidden behind closed doors and avoid going in public just because we have a flare-up. Sometimes we do have to go out in public and there is nothing we can do about it but just hope that the ruddiness isn't showing too much. I have to work every day in an office and meet with clients everyday, so you can imagine that almost on a daily basis I wear a light concealer and SPF combined. Hence when it's time to go out to all these social gatherings, to be honest I'd rather just stay indoors than have to spend time being made to feel uncomfortable.

Yes, sometimes rosacea flares up on one side!

I personally haven't had this experience where rosacea flares on one side of the face and doesn't affect the other side, but I will say that I have seen and read of cases where it does happen. I know of a lady whose rosacea acts up like that. No one quite knows why rosacea does this in some people while it skips others.

For non-rosacea suffers, please be considerate and don't go around asking difficult and insensitive questions that potentially don't have answers. Rosacea is already hard enough to deal with without having the extra burden of people pointing and saying hurtful things. This brings me to my next point, which deals with and tackles the psychological side of rosacea and just how real it is and can be for those suffering from it.

The psychological side of rosacea is real

There are cases of people who have taken their own lives because they could not cope and deal with having to live with rosacea for the rest of their lives. It is sad hearing and reading about such young lives snuffed out in a second because of the pain and the associated emotional stress that often accompanies rosacea sufferers.

The people who normally take their own lives and commit suicide are usually those who have battled rosacea for some time and have found it challenging to go on living for several reasons. These reasons can include people constantly deriding and making fun of them, insensitive remarks, unkind jokes, the list is endless. Sometimes it is just low self-esteem that is accompanied by these hurtful remarks by someone on the outside that pushes a sufferer over the edge and convinces them that they cannot go on living.

The battle in the mind of a person suffering from rosacea is real. This is why I speak passionately to non-rosacea sufferers and advocate for them to be aware of the effect of their words and their actions around rosacea sufferers. Something you may consider small and insignificant can be the last straw that causes someone to lose it. So next time you are about to say something to someone suffering from rosacea, just remember that the psychological battle is very real for rosacea sufferers.

Yes I am eating right and cutting out the stress but rosacea is life long!

Eating right and eating healthily is a recommendation not just for rosacea sufferers but for each and every one of us. When you visit a dermatologist, on your list of recommended treatments and lifestyle changes will be adhering to a well-balanced diet and cutting out food that is both unhealthy and can lead to flare-ups.

You will find that rosacea patients are among some of the people who take better care of their health and who will do anything to make sure that they are healthy. You will find that we not only eat better but we exercise even though after each session we are left feeling very uncomfortable because of the heat on our faces. You will also find that we do our best to cut out all stressful situations as best as we can. When you ask us if we are eating right and cutting out the stress it is a bit insulting considering the great lengths we go to make sure that we have done all those things!

There is still so much that as a non-rosacea patient I wish I could tell you about, but it would make this book too long. The above points are enough to get you started on your journey to be more patient and understanding towards those suffering from rosacea. I hope that these points have opened your eyes to understanding the battles that rosacea patients go through. While this is not a definitive list, it is start that will help you when you are around rosacea patients.

CHAPTER 11 – Final Thoughts

I hope you have found this book full of great tips and advice. You as the rosacea patient play an important part in making sure that the rosacea is kept under control. The following are a few simple final tips to help you on your journey to living life to the fullest while living with rosacea.

Keep a diary

Keeping a journal or diary will help you document what is happening in your life and inadvertently help you chronicle your life with rosacea. You should document how you felt on particular days and what your rosacea was like on those days. With time, you will begin to notice trends and patterns that can give you clues as to when and how your rosacea is triggered.

Perhaps you went out to the beach and enjoyed an afternoon bathing in the sun but when you got home your skin felt like it was on fire and your eyes felt dry. Or perhaps you have had an emotionally stressful week and you noticed that during that week your face was flushing in full force and you found yourself having to use a lot of tinted moisturizer and make-up to cover up the flushing.

Keeping a journal will help you easily identify patterns and habits that tend to trigger the onset of the rosacea. This is a good way to familiarize yourself with the things that trigger rosacea.

Stay out of the sun

We all love warm and sunny days, soaking up some rays, but for us rosacea patients, we need to be careful about how and when we enjoy the sun. Avoid going outside when the sun is at its peak and at its hottest. This obviously depends on where you live geographically but for most places this happens to be midday and in the afternoon.

If you have to be in the sun, make sure you are fully covered and protected by sunscreen with an SPF of 15 and above and that you have an umbrella or a large sunhat that blocks that sun from hitting your face directly.

In general, when summer comes you might have to make a few lifestyle adjustments in order to ensure a pleasant summer experience. If you don't take these necessary proactive steps, you might find yourself having and experiencing more flare-ups than normal.

Avoid too many facial products

This one applies to both men and women. The chemicals used in many facial gels, lotions and creams today can aggravate your rosacea and make it worse. If you have to use make-up and facial creams, look for oil-free make-up and oil-free facial creams. Look for facial creams and make-up that is water-based.

You should also never apply topical steroids to existing rosacea, as this is asking for trouble. You may observe and enjoy temporary relief from your symptoms but in the next weeks after this application you will experience a severe flare-up, which might worsen the rosacea from its current mild state to a more aggressive form.

Also look for products that contain more natural ingredients and not ones with names you can't pronounce.

Always follow and adhere to what your doctors recommend

You will most likely be working with a team of doctors to help you manage and control your rosacea. You may have a dermatologist as your primary doctor, who will be able to give you the best advice when it comes to all things concerning your skin. If you have persistent eye problems, you are going to have to contact an optician or an ophthalmologist. You will need them especially if your eyelids are irritated.

Some people need a therapist. We all know how rosacea can really leave many of us feeling depressed and suffering from low self-esteem. Our appearance is something that is very important to all of us. A scarred appearance can really mess with a person's self-confidence and self-esteem, which can cause them to fall into depression. Other feelings that often accompany rosacea sufferers include feeling embarrassed, frustrated about one's appearance, as well as anger.

So having someone who can help you is very important. People who are entertaining suicidal thoughts will oftentimes need the help of someone else to help them out of their negative self-talk.

Follow a regular Skin Care Regime

One of the most important elements in making sure you stay on top of rosacea is developing a good game plan for your skin care. You need to have a good skin care regime in place to ensure that your skin's needs are well taken care of.

This plan must take into account each and every product that you use on your face, from the soap you use to wash your face, to the cleansers and moisturizers. Each and every one of these products must be carefully selected to make sure that it doesn't contain any irritant substances that will aggravate your skin.

When washing your face you should avoid using hot water, as this can burn your skin as well as be a flare-up trigger. Use lukewarm water on your face. Avoid cold or frigid water as it too can shock your skin. If you wish to test to see if the water is right for your face, you can use your elbow to check.

One last point to make about your skin care regime – ditch the facials, you probably don't need them anyway.

Eliminate Stress from your Life

Whether it is family-related stress or work stress, the bottom line is this - the stress needs to go. Rosacea and stress do not go well together and so you need to prioritize and find a way to cut out the stress in your life.

This isn't always easy, as the stress might be a situation that is beyond your control. For example, if you are the president of a country the way Bill Clinton was, there is no way to get out of such a stressful position, but there are ways to help cut down and reduce the stress.

You might not be able to completely get rid of the stress but you can help bring it down as best as you can. For example, make a to-do list of things you need to cover and achieve each morning as you get into your office. Leave your emails till mid-morning or delegate an assistant to go through them and sort them out for you.

Do the important things first and leave all the minor things for last. Engage in activities that will help you relax on a daily basis such as meditation or exercise.

Avoid Triggers

Every person has a unique set of triggers that affect them primarily. What affects one person may not necessarily be a problem for the next person. As stated above, keeping a diary or a journal will help you track your triggers and help you easily identify them.

Once you have identified your triggers, it then becomes so much easier to avoid them. Personally my triggers include the sun, wind, spicy food and when I use skin care products that contain chemicals I can't even pronounce! These are my own personal triggers.

It took me about a month of carefully detailing all my flare-ups before I could finally say what my triggers were. Sometimes I found out that something I thought was a trigger was not actually a trigger. So it takes a bit of effort to understand your own set of triggers but it becomes worth it in the long run as once you know them, you can easily avoid those things before you subject yourself to the pain of a flare-up.

Use Make-up Only When Needed

Personally I have never been very obsessed with make-up but I am aware of people who cannot live without it. With that said, I found it important to include this tip in here for them.

Make-up in and of itself is not wrong and is not to be avoided completely. When it comes to using make-up as a rosacea patient, you have to treat it like all other potential triggers; you have to use it with caution and sparingly. Only use it when necessary and use the right products on your face.

We have spoken in depth about the different make-up ingredients you should avoid and use in several places in this book, but in a nutshell, look for a BB or CC cream as these creams will combine coverage products and provide an SPF all in one product. You don't want to be applying five different products on your face every day so a BB cream will be best.

When looking for powders or primers, look for yellow tinted ones that come in mineral powder form. Also look for products that do not contain essential oils in them such as rose and peppermint.

Stay Hydrated

Keeping your skin hydrated does a world of good for you. It keeps your skin looking soft and supple as well as helping to keep you cool. Hydration products are worth looking out for, especially in your facial cleansers and moisturizers. Look out for products that contain Aloe Vera, Chamomile and Cucumber. The more natural you go the better.

Remembering to drink plenty of water a day is also a good way to ensure that you are well hydrated. If you engage in physical activity or exercise, this is an even better reason to make sure that you keep yourself well hydrated, as you are raising your body's temperature and are more likely to suffer flare-ups after your session is over.

Drink water continually throughout your exercise to help keep you cool and also make sure that you exercise underneath a fan to help you get rid of the extra heat as and when you workout.

These are some of the top tips that I use when I am working out and in my day–to-day life. I hope that you will incorporate them into your daily life. Try and incorporate at least one new tip every week so that you can work actively to get your rosacea under control.

Good news for Rosacea patients - there is research being carried out

Teams of medical doctors, particularly in the United States. are actively involved in the research of rosacea, its causes and effects. The areas of interest that are being tackled actively involve:

- The development of new medicine that will help fight the effects of rosacea
- Gaining a better understanding on just how the body's immune system is affected by rosacea
- How to reduce the amount of scarring that takes place when extra skin tissue is removed from swollen noses
- How to effectively combat and overcome the eye problems that are affecting Rosacea patients.

The fight against rosacea is being fought in the labs, as progress is made and we try to understand more about rosacea. Rosacea might be incurable today, but there might be a cure soon in the not-to-distant future!

CHAPTER 12 – Frequently Asked Questions

Q. What is Seborrheic Dermatitis?

A. Seborrheic Dermatitis, often shortened to seb derm, is one of the most common conditions of the skin that affect rosacea sufferers. It appears at similar times with rosacea. Medical experts say that the two skin ailments are unrelated. The National Rosacea Society of America estimates that at least one quarter of diagnosed rosacea patients also have seborrheic dermatitis. A common and effective seb derm treatment is 25% zinc pryrithione cream applied up to three times a day.

Q. My Rosacea symptoms appear in winter only. Is it possible to have 'winter rosacea'?

A. What will affect one rosacea patient might not always affect the next rosacea patient. A good example of this is seborrheic dermatitis or rhinoplasty. Not every rosacea patient is affected by every single symptom of the condition. For some their rosacea is mild, for others the symptoms are moderate. For some the symptoms like in your case appear and flare-up in one particular season. What this probably means is that your skin is simply more sensitive to the wind and cold weather than other patients.

Q. What causes rosacea?

A. Medical doctors are still not sure just what causes rosacea. There are several theories about what might be the cause such as blood vessels in the face that easily dilate bring blood to the surface of the skin, making the skin look flushed.

There are also environmental factors that may trigger rosacea symptoms such as change in seasons but these are not what cause rosacea.

Q. Is rosacea contagious?

A. Medically speaking, rosacea is not classified as a contagious disease. Because rosacea is not caused by a virus or bacteria it cannot be transmitted by physical contact or via airborne means.

Q. Is rosacea hereditary?

A. There is no evidence that supports the assumption that rosacea is hereditary to date. There have been no experiments done to test the theory that rosacea is hereditary. However, this does not remove the evidence that points to the fact that rosacea may be hereditary. Up to 40 percent of patients that participated in a survey by the American National Rosacea Society have found a genetic link between themselves and a relative with the same condition.

When looking at issues of ethnicity in another survey conducted by the American National Rosacea Society again, the survey showed that more than 33 percent of participants who had rosacea had one Irish parent and close to 26 percent had one parent who was of English descent. Rosacea when compared among ethnicities was seen as being generally higher in those who carried Welsh, Scottish or Scandinavian heritage.

Q. How do you test for rosacea?

A. A general physician can check for rosacea by making a careful observation of the symptoms you exhibit. This checkup and a look into your medical history can help the physician determine what they believe to be the cause of the symptoms you exhibit and hence give a proper diagnosis.

In the event that you are referred to a dermatologist, they can further run a few tests that include taking a biopsy to eliminate other similar conditions. Make sure to give the physician or dermatologist as accurate a rundown of your symptoms as possible.

Q. Does rosacea get worse with time?

A. Age and time make no difference to the general condition of your rosacea as long as you are on a regular treatment program. What does make a difference however is your consistency in keeping up with your therapy and avoiding the triggers that are specific to you. It is a well-documented fact that those who are inconsistent with their rosacea treatment tend to suffer worse flare-ups than those who maintain and keep to their prescribed medication and lifestyle that avoids their rosacea triggers. Age doesn't make your rosacea any worse or any better – it's how you manage and adhere to your treatment options that does.

Q. Will my rosacea ever end?

A. Sadly rosacea is known as a chronic illness, which means that it has far reaching effects and will likely continue. Rosacea has no known cure but there are ways to minimize its effect and reach. If successfully managed, you can go on living your life normally and suffer the occasional flare-up here and there but nothing too dramatic. So the two main things to remember about managing rosacea are: one, adhere to your prescribed rosacea treatment and two, look into your lifestyle and make the necessary changes that will enable you to live as normal a life as possible without regular flare-ups.

Q. Where do I find a rosacea doctor?

A. The world that we live in has now become so technologically advanced that there is almost nothing and no one you can't find online. If you are looking for a 'rosacea doctor' then you probably won't find one. What you need to do is search for a good dermatologist online. Generally dermatologists are the specialist doctors you should be going to when you are worried about rosacea. Dermatologists are doctors who have specialized in issues that affect the skin, hair and nails, so they are most likely able to give advice on the best treatment options for rosacea. If you have a general physician that you go to often, ask them for a referral to a good dermatologist.

Q. Should I be worried that my children will get rosacea if I have it?

A. Rosacea can occur and affect your children years later. There isn't a lot of evidence to conclusively state that rosacea is hereditary, although there is some evidence that seems to point in that direction. The long and short of the answer is yes, there is a possibility that your children might suffer from rosacea after you. If you are worried that your future children might be rosacea patients or that your existing children might be at risk, all you need to do for now is keep an eye open for the telltale symptoms. The sooner you catch rosacea, the sooner you can get a treatment option in place.

Q. Where can I find a support group?

A. The leading support organization in the world for all things rosacea is the American National Rosacea Society. Their website rosacea.org is a great tool that is full of rich teachings and articles that are specifically aimed at rosacea patients. You will find great help from the website, as I have done over the years. It is one website that I enjoy visiting to find out the truth about a certain topic.

In the event that you are looking for more personal forums, you will be able to find these on the different search engines by simply typing in 'rosacea patient chat groups and forums'. Two places that will give you a head start are rosacea-support.org and yahoogroups.com. You will find online forums and chat groups from these two resources.

Q. My skin feels very hot during a flare-up, why does it get so hot?

A. This is one of the telltale symptoms of rosacea. This happens for two major reasons. The first reason is that this may be the body's reaction to an outward stimulus such as the sun or a harsh facial product. The second reason may be that the body's temperature has increased. In order to eliminate and get rid of this excessive heat, the blood vessels in the body (the face especially) must dilate to increase blood flow towards the skin. This allows the heat to escape via the skin, permitting the body's temperature to go back to normal. As this heat leaves your body via the skin, the temperature of your skin will increase. This is why when you touch your skin during a flare-up you will discover that it feels warm to the touch. The reason you see the redness is because of the dilated blood vessels which become slightly visible underneath the skin, hence the ruddiness.

Q. I have read about staying clear of 'harsh facial products' but just what should I be looking out for in these products?

A. The sensitive nature of rosacea patients' skin means you need to avoid facial cleansers or products that contain allergens or flare-up triggers such as perfumes, color additives, and alcohol. The products you should be choosing as a rosacea patient need to contain key natural ingredients such as chamomile, aloe vera, cucumber and green tea. This is because each of these products is perfect for sensitive skin and skin that has potential redness issues such as ours. These ingredients serve to soothe, bring about a cooling effect while hydrating the skin. Other products that you should avoid are essential oils like Lanolin, Arnica, Peppermint, Witch Hazel and Rose.

Q. I am worried about using foundation, concealer and SPF together. Won't they cause my skin to flare-up big time?

A. The truth of the matter is that yes, every product you apply to your face has the potential of being a trigger. However, this does not mean you will never wear make-up again. The trick to wearing make-up when you are a rosacea sufferer is to remember that less is more. Mineral-based products are your best bet and so are yellow tinted powders and primers. You will read about people talking about green tinted make-up helping to cover the redness, I don't disagree with that but the only problem that I find with green tinted make-up is that it leaves your face looking a bit grey. I find that yellow based products are much, much better. The best way that I have found to wear make-up without using too many products is to find a BB or CC cream that incorporates elements of coverage, other healthy skin care needs and sun protection all into one product. These kinds of creams really help in cutting down the number of products you apply to your face.

Q. How is Rosacea different from Acne?

A. This has got to be the number one asked question at the start of every rosacea patient's journey, particularly when you are still looking for an answer to, 'Will it ever end?' Acne as we know generally starts during your pubescent years and should end as you reach your twenties. Rosacea on the other hand normally starts towards your late twenties, or thirties and sometimes even when one is older and sadly never comes to an end. The main difference between the two is firstly the time they begin to appear and also the symptoms they exhibit.

Pimples that are caused by acne are often found below the skin and are linked to bacteria. The common acne symptoms are black heads, white heads, and the occasional pustule. With Rosacea on the other hand, you discover that you have the same bumps but this time they are found directly on the skin and can also affect the nose as well as the eyes. The treatment methods of the two conditions are also very different.

Hence getting the right diagnosis from the onset is very crucial and important in your fight against rosacea.

Q. What are FDA approved treatments that I can use?

FDA treatments or medication refers to drugs that have been tested under the strictest conditions in American laboratories and checked for any potentially harmful elements by the Food and Drug Administration. When a drug, gel or food has passed this rigorous testing it is given the green light and can be sold on the market freely. Examples of FDA approved medications for rosacea include:

Oracea, which is a doxycycline pill that is used to effectively bring down rosacea-related bumps

Soolantra, which is 1% ivermectin cream, works in much the same way as Oracea in that it helps to significantly reduce rosacea related red pimples

Mirvaso is the only FDA topical gel that has received the green light to be sold on the market. It helps reduce the ruddiness of rosacea.

All of these medications can be found in pharmacies across the country or bought from regulated online stores.

Q. I heard someone say there are different types of rosacea, is this true?

A. Yes, there are four different types of rosacea. The four groups that are commonly agreed upon are erythematotelangiectatic, ocular rosacea, phymatous, and papulopustular. Each one is different from the other and showcases a different set of symptoms. Each one of these rosacea types can be identified by your dermatologist. In doing this you will also be able to get the correct treatment to help fix your problem. While they do have and share common rosacea symptoms, they are all independent and their effects need to be carefully monitored so that a specific program tailored for you can be devised by your dermatologist. Keeping a journal or diary of your flare-ups can also help your doctor out when he or she is trying to determine which type of rosacea you have.

Conclusion

There is no doubt that having rosacea is anything but easy. It will come about at the most inopportune times and then suddenly be less apparent. The bottom line is that you have to figure out what triggers it and keep it at bay. I know that it's a constant struggle to live with this issue, but if you know how to deal with it properly, you have already won half the battle.

Regardless of what age you get rosacea at, you can manage the symptoms and learn how to continue living your life as normally as possible. We have mentioned all the symptoms you may experience during the condition. In addition, we have also discussed what the most commons causes for flare-ups are. Of course, keep in mind that these will differ from person to person. However, it's vital to know them all just to be on the safe side.

So starting today, stop living life in hiding. Instead, it's time to come out of the shadows and show people the true you. This book will help you do just that. I wish you the best of luck, from one rosacea sufferer to another

Resources

Important: the websites mentioned in this book were all active at the time of printing, As the Internet changes rapidly, it might be that these websites are no longer active, This, of course, is out of my control.

FORUMS AND FORUMS AND CHAT GROUPS
www.irosacea.org

www.yahoogroups.com

www.rosacea-support.org

WEBSITES

www.aad.org (American Academy of Dermatology)

www.niams.nih.gov/Health_Info/Rosacea/rosacea_ff.asp

www.rosacea.org

www.rosacea.org/patients/allaboutrosacea.php

Mayo Clinic

www.dermnetnz.org/acne/rosacea.html

www.bad.org.uk/for-the-public/patient-information-leaflets/rosacea (British Association of Dermatologists)

www.irosacea.org/index.html (The Rosacea Research & Development Institute)

www.emedicine.medscape.com/article/1071429-overview

www.rosaceaguide.com

Make-up related websites

Voices.yahoo.com

http://www.bodyandsoul.com.au

http://www.totalbeauty.com

http://makeup.lovetoknow.com

http://www.sheknows.com

Published by IMB Publishing 2015

Copyright and Trademarks: This publication is Copyrighted 2015 by IMB Publishing. All products, publications, software and services mentioned and recommended in this publication are protected by trademarks. In such instance, all trademarks & copyright belong to the respective owners. All rights reserved. No part of this book may be reproduced or transferred in any form or by any means, graphic, electronic, or mechanical, including photocopying, recording, taping, or by any information storage retrieval system, without the written permission of the authors. Pictures used in this book are either royalty free pictures bought from stock-photo websites or have the source mentioned underneath the picture.

Disclaimer and Legal Notice: This product is not legal or medical advice and should not be interpreted in that manner. You need to do your own due-diligence to determine if the content of this product is right for you. The authors and the affiliates of this product are not liable for any damages or losses associated with the content in this product. While every attempt has been made to verify the information shared in this publication, neither the author nor the affiliates assume any responsibility for errors, omissions or contrary interpretation of the subject matter herein. Any perceived slights to any specific person(s) or organization(s) are purely unintentional. We have no control over the nature, content and availability of the web sites listed in this book.

The inclusion of any web site links does not necessarily imply a recommendation or endorse the views expressed within them. IMB Publishing takes no responsibility for, and will not be liable for, the websites being temporarily unavailable or being removed from the Internet.

The accuracy and completeness of information provided herein and opinions stated herein are not guaranteed or warranted to produce any particular results, and the advice and strategies, contained herein may not be suitable for every individual. The author shall not be liable for any loss incurred as a consequence of the use and application, directly or indirectly, of any information presented in this work. This publication is designed to provide information in regard to the subject matter covered.

The information included in this book has been compiled to give an overview of the subject and detail some of the symptoms, treatments etc. that are available. It is not intended to give medical advice. For a firm diagnosis of any health condition, and for a treatment plan suitable for you and your dog, you should consult your veterinarian or consultant.

The writer of this book and the publisher are not responsible for any damages or negative consequences following any of the treatments or methods highlighted in this book. Website links are for informational purposes and should not be seen as a personal endorsement; the same applies to the products detailed in this book. The reader should also be aware that although the web links included were correct at the time of writing, they may become out of date in the future.